Management of Infertility for the MRCOG and Beyond

Third edition

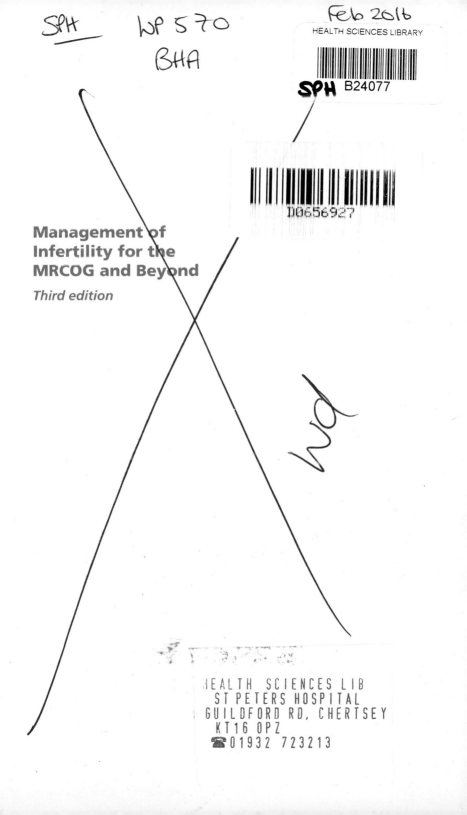

Management of Infertility for the MRCOG and Beyond

Third edition

Edited by Siladitya Bhattacharya and Mark Hamilton

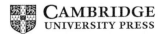

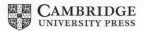

Cambridge, New York, Melbourne, Madrid, Cape Town, Singapore, São Paulo, Delhi, Mexico City

Cambridge University Press
The Edinburgh Building, Cambridge CB2 8RU, UK

Published in the United States of America by Cambridge University Press, New York

www.cambridge.org
Information on this title: www.cambridge.org/9781107678576

First published 2014

Printed and bound in the United Kingdom by Bell and Bain Ltd

A catalogue record for this publication is available from the British Library

ISBN 978-1-107-67857-6 Paperback

Contents

About the authors

Siladitya Bhattacharya MBBS MD MRCOG
Head of Division of Applied Health Sciences, School of Medicine & Dentistry, University of Aberdeen, Aberdeen Maternity Hospital, Cornhill Road, Aberdeen AB25 2ZD

Kirsty Brookes MBChB MRCOG
Specialist Registrar in Obstetrics and Gynaecology, Salisbury District Hospital, Odstock Road, Salisbury SP2 8BJ

Ying Cheong MBChB BAO MA MD MRCOG
Senior Lecturer and Honorary Consultant in Obstetrics and Gynaecology, Academic Unit of Human Development and Health, Faculty of Medicine, University of Southampton, Southampton SO16 6YD

Tim Child MA MD MRCOG
University of Oxford, Oxford Fertility Unit, Institute of Reproductive Sciences, Oxford Business Park North, Oxford OX4 2HW

Mark Hamilton MD FRCOG
Department of Obstetrics and Gynaecology, University of Aberdeen, Aberdeen Maternity Hospital, Foresterhill, Aberdeen AB25 2ZL

Haitham Hamoda MD MRCOG
Consultant Gynaecologist, Subspecialist in Reproductive Medicine and Surgery, King's College Hospital, Denmark Hill, London SE5 9RS

Yacoub Khalaf MD FRCOG MFFP
Consultant Gynaecologist & Clinical Director, The Assisted Conception Unit & Centre for Pre-implantation Genetic Diagnosis, 11th Floor, Tower Wing, Guy's Hospital, London SE1 9RT

Abha Maheshwari MD MRCOG
Department of Obstetrics and Gynaecology, University of Aberdeen, Aberdeen Maternity Hospital, Foresterhill, Aberdeen AB25 2ZL

Neil McClure MD FRCOG
Queen's University Belfast, Mulhouse Building, Grosvenor Road, Belfast BT12 6DP

Srividya Seshadri MD MRCOG
Sub-specialist Registrar in Reproductive Medicine and Surgery, The Assisted Conception Unit & Centre for Pre-implantation Genetic Diagnosis, 11th Floor, Tower Wing, Guy's Hospital, London SE1 9RT

Jane Stewart BSc MBChB MD FRCOG
Newcastle Fertility Centre at Life, Biomedicine West Wing, International Centre for Life, Times Square, Newcastle upon Tyne NE1 4EP

Preface

Infertility affects up to one in six couples and remains a major cause of distress in both men and women. Concerns about fertility continue to grow across the world along with economic and social pressures causing women to delay childbirth, and the impact of lifestyle factors such as obesity, smoking and alcohol intake.

The last two decades have witnessed a shift towards evidence-based fertility treatment and greater awareness of the need to ensure the highest standards of safety. Management of infertility has moved away from an aetiological pathway where physicians identify and then treat an underlying pathology, to a prognostic approach where the decision to initiate treatment is driven by awareness of a couple's chances of spontaneous conception and what can be achieved with intervention.

To address the changes in the way fertility problems are now diagnosed, investigated and managed, we have substantially redesigned the third edition of this book, enlisting a new cast of authors and expanding the scope of the text. While the evidence base underpinning the choice of tests and treatments is sometimes far from secure, clinical decisions should be made jointly with patients and should maximise health gains while minimising costs and risks.

Infertility remains an integral part of core training for those taking the MRCOG examination. We hope that this book will provide a concise guide to fertility practice for trainees as well as for specialists.

Siladitya Bhattacharya and Mark Hamilton
2013

Acknowledgements

We would like to thank all the authors for their contributions and Claire Dunn for her patience. We also owe an enormous debt of gratitude to Margery Heath, without whose efforts this book would not have been completed.

Abbreviations

AFC	antral follicle count
AMH	antimüllerian hormone
ART	assisted reproductive technology
AZF	azoospermia factor
CBAVD	congenital bilateral absence of the vas deferens
cGMP	cyclic guanosine monophosphate
BMI	body mass index
DHT	dihydrotestosterone
FSH	follicle-stimulating hormone
GnRH	gonadotrophin-releasing hormone
hCG	human chorionic gonadotrophin
HFEA	Human Fertilisation and Embryology Authority
hMG	human menopausal gonadotrophin
HP-FSH	highly purified FSH
HPV	human papillomavirus
HRT	hormone replacement therapy
HSG	hysterosalpingography/hysterosalpingogram
HyCoSy	hysterosalpingo-contrast-sonography
ICSI	intracytoplasmic sperm injection
IUCD	intrauterine contraceptive device
IUI	intrauterine insemination
IVF	in vitro fertilisation
JZ	junctional zone
LH	luteinising hormone
LHRH	luteinising hormone-releasing hormone
M/ml	million per millilitre
MRI	magnetic resonance imaging
NICE	National Institute for Health and Care Excellence
OHSS	ovarian hyperstimulation syndrome
OR	odds ratio
PCOS	polycystic ovary syndrome
PCT	postcoital test
PGD	pre-implantation genetic diagnosis
PGS	pre-implantation genetic screening
RCT	randomised controlled trial
SHBG	sex hormone-binding globulin

SIS	saline infusion sonography
SO	superovulation
SSRI	selective serotonin reuptake inhibitor
STI	sexually transmitted infection
TSH	thyroid-stimulating hormone
TVUS	transvaginal ultrasound
UAE	uterine artery embolisation
VEGF	vascular endothelial growth factor
WHO	World Health Organization

1 Epidemiology and initial assessment

Introduction

This chapter discusses the prevalence of infertility and the importance of the initial assessment of the infertile couple. Efficient mechanisms for referral and investigation and adoption of region-wide protocols of basic investigation are requirements for those involved in the planning of services, and should be founded upon good liaison between medical and nursing staff in both primary and secondary care. Adherence to such protocols facilitates appropriate and timely investigation along standardised paths, minimising the risks of delay and repetition of tests, which couples find particularly demoralising. Once a diagnosis is reached, it should be possible to offer the infertile couple an accurate prognosis and the opportunity to consider the issues relevant to treatment choices for their particular situation.

Epidemiology

A common definition of infertility is the inability of a couple to conceive following 12–24 months of exposure to pregnancy. The length of exposure time considered is determined by the observation that in the general population, which would include a proportion of couples with infertility, one would expect the chance of conception in any individual cycle to be around 20%. Thus by 1 year of exposure about 85% of couples would have achieved conception and by the time 2 years has elapsed some 92% would have conceived. In practical terms, the failure to achieve pregnancy causes enormous distress to those affected. For people with fertility problems, using a definition of 1 year to describe infertility is usual and most will have sought medical advice or assistance by that time.

Natural fertility rates decline in association with increasing female age, although in an ultimately fertile group of women it is not certain that their monthly fecundity rate (chance of conception) is any less than that in younger cohorts. It may be sensible to consider specialist referral of women over the age of 35 years in advance of 1 year. However, it should be recognised that in many instances conception will occur naturally in these cases, since it can be assumed that a proportion will not be infertile.

Estimates of the prevalence of infertility in the population are influenced by the duration of infertility used in the definition and by the setting of the population studied, for example primary care or hospital clinics. Community-based data will give an accurate reflection of prevalence within the general population but are limited. Published prevalence studies show a range of lifetime risk of infertility varying from 6.6% to 32.6%. One population-based study in the north-east of Scotland, which also took account of conceptions resulting in miscarriage and ectopic pregnancy, found a prevalence of 14% using a 2-year definition.

A number of factors have been a matter of concern in recent years with respect to their potential impact on the prevalence of infertility, including the incidence of sexually transmitted infections (STIs) such as *Chlamydia trachomatis* in the young. In addition, there have been suggestions that environmental factors may affect male fertility. Profound questions have also been raised about the effects on female fertility of delayed childbearing as a result of changes in lifestyle and working patterns. Despite these legitimate concerns, when the population-based study was repeated, the observed prevalence of infertility had not increased in north-east Scotland in the succeeding 20 years.

A lack of observed change in prevalence should not encourage complacency in respect of public health responsibilities. Opportunities to prevent infertility are limited, and encouraging young people to engage in safe sexual practices that limit exposure to risk of STIs is clearly important. For teenage girls, rubella immunisation programmes should be in place. Human papillomavirus (HPV) vaccination programmes are now being established. Education of the public about the known decline in fertility that occurs with age, particularly in women older than 35 years, is also important. Furthermore, folic acid supplementation for women to reduce the risk of neural tube defects should be promoted, as should making certain lifestyle adjustments such as reducing smoking and alcohol consumption and achieving optimal weight. There is convincing evidence that smoking, whether active or passive, affects reproductive performance in both women and men, and that it increases the risks in pregnancy of small-for-gestational-age infants, stillbirth and infant mortality.

Initial assessment

PRIMARY CARE

The role of the GP is crucial. Infertility represents a deeply personal problem and many people would prefer to discuss intimate matters with someone they know and trust. The support that the GP can provide in terms of counselling and preliminary investigations is an excellent foundation for provision of care. Not infrequently, the man and woman may be registered with different GPs. One should always consider that infertility is a problem affecting both parties and each may contribute to the pathogenesis. Once referral is made to a specialist clinic, the stresses imposed on couples may increase, with demands on their time for attendance, the indignity of some of the investigations carried out and the invasion of privacy that occurs. Since it is well recognised that infertility investigation and treatment pose real threats to domestic stability, it is the GP, through knowledge of the couple and their families, who may be in the best position to provide support for those struggling to come to terms with continued disappointment.

All patients should be seen as couples in appropriate surroundings. Facilities should be available to permit examination of both partners and sufficient time, usually half an hour, should be set aside to make an adequate overall assessment of the problem.

It may be helpful for the local fertility clinic to employ dedicated liaison staff to assist with the referral process and with guideline dissemination. In some instances, tubal assessment might be organised in primary care, although before committing to intrusive investigation it would be wise to have information on semen quality beforehand. This can be difficult where the male partner has a different GP to the female but improved communication within primary care can resolve this issue. Bearing in mind the statutory requirement in offering licensed treatment to take account of the welfare of the potential child or existing children, it is essential that GPs give this some thought at this early stage to avoid difficulties in later management.

HOSPITAL CARE

Hospital care should be provided in a setting under the clinical direction of a consultant gynaecologist with a special interest in infertility. Patients should be seen in a dedicated fertility clinic with appropriate appointment times to permit thorough evaluation. A team system should be established involving medical, nursing, laboratory (endocrine and andrology) and counselling personnel to facilitate a consistent and coordinated approach to care. The level of treatment options available will depend on the expertise of, and the facilities available to, staff at each centre.

The infertility consultation

The point at which any couple might seek assistance will be influenced by a number of factors, not least the degree of anxiety that couples feel in confronting seemingly relentless monthly disappointments. Any couple worried about their fertility should thus be seen by their GP, regardless of the duration of their infertility. It is unusual for couples to present if this is less than a year but it may be apparent to individuals that they may be at risk of a fertility problem and they seek advice at an early stage. For example, the man may have had a vasectomy or undergone testicular surgery in childhood such as orchidopexy; either partner may be a survivor of childhood cancer and have undergone chemotherapy; or the woman may be aware of an association of absent or irregular periods with infertility. For some, a concern through the high profile that infertility now has in the media may have eroded self-assurance about personal fecundity. Unless there is a clear need on the basis of history or examination of either partner, further investigation is usually unnecessary if the duration of infertility is less than 1 year. Providing the couple with an outline of their excellent potential fertility may be all that is required to set their minds at rest. However, couples who present early may themselves have particular concerns or have problems that merit sympathetic discussion. A little more urgency may also be required in the investigation of couples where the female partner is over 35 years of age.

Three simple questions need to be addressed in the assessment of an infertile couple:

1 Are sperm available? (Is there evidence of normal sperm production and ejaculatory competence?)
2 Are eggs available? (Is the woman ovulating?)
3 Can the gametes meet? (Is female pelvic anatomy normal and is coital function adequate?)

The steps in the process of investigating infertility should be discussed at the outset with the couple in the expectation that all necessary tests would be complete within 4 months. The sequence with which tests are performed is, to some extent, standardised for all but may vary if history or examination findings suggest otherwise. Initial investigations are inexpensive, non-invasive and likely to yield useful information.

Points requiring particular attention in the history and examination of the couple are shown in Tables 1.1 and 1.2.

A psychological assessment of the impact of perceived infertility on individuals and the couple is an essential component of this initial encounter. Libido and consequently coital frequency may be profoundly influenced by the experience of infertility and thus affect prognosis.

Preliminary investigations

FEMALE

At the outset, it is advisable to ensure that the woman is rubella immune and that she is taking folic acid (0.4 mg/day) to reduce the chance of the fetus developing a neural tube defect. There may be particular circumstances where a higher dose of folic acid (5 mg/day) is recommended, such as in women taking anti-epileptic medication, those who are obese (with a body mass index [BMI] above 30 kg/m^2), when either partner or a previous child has a neural tube defect, or women with diabetes, coeliac disease or thalassaemia.

The preliminary investigation centres on the need to demonstrate that the woman is ovulating. This is almost certainly the case if she has a regular monthly cycle. Laboratory evidence may be obtained through measurement of serum progesterone in the putative luteal phase of the menstrual cycle. Levels should

Table 1.1 **The initial assessment of female infertility: history and examination**

Area of investigation	History
Infertility	• Duration of infertility • Duration and type of contraceptive use • Fertility in previous relationships as well as in current liaison • Previous investigation and treatment • Fertility subsequently, if known, in any former partners • Previous fertility investigations and treatment

Medical	• Menstrual history:
	  o menarche
	  o cycle length and duration of flow
	  o pain
	  o bouts of amenorrhoea
	  o menorrhagia
	  o intermenstrual bleeding
	• Number of previous pregnancies, including terminations of pregnancy, miscarriages and ectopic pregnancies
	• Any associated sepsis
	• STIs
	• Time to initiate previous pregnancies
	• Drug history past and present, such as agents that cause hyperprolactinaemia, past cytotoxic treatment or radiotherapy

Surgical	• Previous abdominal or pelvic surgery, in particular gynaecological procedures
Occupational	• Work patterns, including separation from partner
Sexual	• Coital frequency and timing, including knowledge of the fertile period • Dyspareunia • Postcoital bleeding
Area of investigation	Examination
General	• Height, weight, BMI • Fat and hair distribution (Ferriman–Gallwey score to quantify hirsutism) • Note presence or absence of acne and galactorrhoea
Abdominal	• Check for abdominal masses or tenderness
Pelvis	• Assess state of hymen • Assess normality of clitoris and labia • Assess vagina, looking for problems such as infection, a vaginal septum or endometriotic deposits • Check for presence of cervical polyps • Assess accessibility of the cervix for insemination • Record uterine size, position, mobility and tenderness • Perform cervical smear if appropriate

BMI = body mass index; STIs = sexually transmitted infections

be in excess of 30 nmol/l 7 days after ovulation. For this reason, sampling should be arranged for day 21 in the context of a 28-day cycle, with serial checks made beyond this point if the cycle is more prolonged or variable in length. Results

Table 1.2 The initial assessment of male infertility: history and examination

Area of investigation	History
Infertility	• Duration of infertility • Fertility in previous relationships as well as in current liaison • Fertility subsequently, if known, in any former partners • Previous fertility investigations and treatment
Medical	• STIs • Epididymitis • Mumps orchitis • Testicular maldescent • Chronic disease • Drug/alcohol abuse • Recent febrile illness • Recurrent urinary tract infection
Surgical	• Herniorrhaphy • Testicular injury • Torsion • Orchidopexy • Vasectomy (and reversal)
Occupational	• Toxic substance exposure, including chemicals, and radiation exposure • Time away from home through work
Sexual	• Onset of puberty • Coital habits • Premature ejaculation • Libido/impotence • Use and knowledge of the fertile period
Area of investigation	*Examination*
General	• Height, weight, BMI • Fat and hair distribution • Evidence of hypoandrogenism or gynaecomastia
Groin	• Exclude inguinal hernia (patient in upright position) • Check for inguinal mass, such as ectopic testicle
Genitalia	• Note site of testicles in the scrotum and measure volume using an orchidometer • Palpate epididymis for nodularity or tenderness • Check presence and normality of the vasa deferentia • Check for the presence of a varicocele • Examine penis for any structural abnormality, such as hypospadias

BMI = body mass index; STIs = sexually transmitted infections

should be interpreted only in relation to the onset of the subsequent period. If the level is below 30 nmol/l, the test should be repeated in a subsequent cycle. In the absence of any clues in history or examination to suggest the possibility of an endocrine disorder, these tests would be sufficient. If, however, there is a history of irregular menstruation, or periods of amenorrhoea (particularly if associated with galactorrhoea, hirsutism or obesity), then additional biochemical tests are appropriate. This might include measurements of thyroid function, prolactin, and androgen production. This is discussed further in Chapter 3. Robust evidence is lacking to suggest that the use of temperature charts and luteinising hormone (LH) detection methods to time intercourse increases the chance of conception and the routine use of these should be discouraged.

MALE

Semen analysis remains the most important means of assessment. It is desirable, to avoid unhelpful and frustrating duplication, for GP referred assessments to take place in the same laboratory that serves the clinic to which the couple may ultimately be referred. Clear instructions on the provision of samples should be given – a period of abstinence of at least 3 days but no longer than 1 week is desirable, and the sample should be kept at body temperature during transportation and should arrive at the laboratory if being provided off-site within 1 hour of production. In most instances, if the result is normal, a single sample will suffice. If an abnormality is found then the sample should be repeated, usually after at least 1 month to minimise anxiety levels for the man, particularly in cases of azoospermia. Taking account of the biology of sperm production (Chapter 2), it should be borne in mind that resolution of any transient insult leading to defects in sperm production may not be apparent for up to 3 months.

What constitutes a normal result is a matter of debate. Large laboratories may have their own local population-based reference ranges but, in the absence of local information, the World Health Organization (WHO) expected range of values in a fertile population can be applied. These were updated in 2010 and the lower reference limits are shown in Table 1.3. The use of these lower limits as predictors of pregnancy is poor. More complex tests of sperm function, including their potential for movement, cervical mucus penetration, capacitation, zona recognition, the acrosome reaction and sperm–oocyte fusion, have been developed but in practice

Table 1.3 Laboratory reference ranges for semen characteristics

Semen parameter	Lower reference limit (5th centile and its 95% confidence interval)
Semen volume (ml)	1.5 (1.4–1.7)
Total sperm number ($\times 10^6$ per ejaculate)	39 (33–46)
Sperm concentration ($\times 10^6$ per ml)	15 (12–16)
Total motility (progressive and non-progressive, %)	40 (38–42)
Progressive motility (%)	32 (31–34)
Sperm morphology (normal forms, %)	4 (3.0–4.0)

Source: World Health Organization (2010) *WHO Laboratory Manual for the Examination and Processing of Human Semen.* 5th ed. Geneva: WHO.

are rarely required. Further detailed discussion of the assessment and treatment of male factor infertility is given in Chapter 2.

The investigations outlined above can be initiated by the GP but they also provide the basis for hospital investigation. It may be helpful to send the couple a questionnaire to supplement the information provided in the GP's referral letter. Valuable time can be saved if progesterone monitoring, rubella assessment, chlamydia screening and semen analysis are performed in line with current guidelines before referral to the fertility clinic.

In the fertility clinic setting, a pelvic ultrasound examination may be useful. It may reveal potentially significant pathology such as fibroids, intrauterine polyps or ovarian cysts that might be missed in bimanual pelvic examination. Screening tests for bacterial vaginosis and chlamydia should be considered in women at risk and particularly in those with symptoms of vaginal discharge or dysmenorrhoea, past history of STIs or pelvic inflammatory disease.

General advice for practitioners to give to patients

Table 1.4 gives a summary of lifestyle advice that health professionals should provide to patients with infertility. There is reasonable evidence that smoking reduces female fertility, while in men it is known that smoking can affect sperm quality. In men there is evidence that high alcohol intake can influence reproductive function adversely, as well as general health. There is less convincing evidence linking alcohol and female fertility, but intake in excess of two units of alcohol per day is thought to be detrimental to the fetus in pregnancy. Women with a BMI in excess of $30 \, kg/m^2$ should be encouraged to lose weight as, in those with disturbed regulation of ovulation, doing so may restore normal function, or alternatively enhance the response to treatment where instituted. Hyperthermia may adversely affect sperm quality.

Table 1.4	Lifestyle advice to be given to patients with infertility
Lifestyle factor	Recommendation
Smoking	Advise both partners to stop smoking
Alcohol	Advise both partners to limit alcohol intake
Body weight	Encourage women with a BMI in excess of $30 \, kg/m^2$ to lose weight
Sexual intercourse	Advise couples to have regular intercourse at least two or three times per week

BMI = body mass index

While there is some evidence that semen parameters may be adversely affected by very frequent ejaculation, the evidence suggests that fertility potential is unaffected. Bearing in mind that sperm survival can be expected for up to 7 days within the female reproductive tract, couples should be advised to have intercourse every 2–3 days to optimise the chance of conception.

Further tests

FEMALE

Where preliminary investigations suggest that the woman is ovulating and sperm production is satisfactory, pelvic assessment should be considered. For women with symptoms of painful periods or examination findings suggestive of pelvic pathology, laparoscopy and dye hydrotubation will be the investigation of choice. Endometriosis and peritubal adhesions may be found. Hysterosalpingography (HSG) is a simpler test and may be used as a first-line examination in those where there is lower index of suspicion. Tubal assessment should not be carried out if the woman is menstruating. In addition, women should be advised to avoid conception in the cycle in which the procedure is carried out. If unprotected intercourse has occurred then the examination should be deferred.

It is debatable whether assessment of tubal status is necessary in other clinical situations, particularly in women with long-standing, otherwise unexplained, infertility. Current evidence would suggest that minor abnormalities of the uterine cavity such as tubocornual polyps are of little importance in the genesis of infertility. The use of ultrasound in combination with sonoreflective contrast media to visualise intrauterine and tubal pathology has in the last two decades emerged as an alternative outpatient investigation.

Prospective studies are also awaited to determine whether hysteroscopy may have a part to play in the routine investigation of infertile women, although in women with identified intrauterine abnormalities hysteroscopic surgery may be feasible. Women considered at risk, generally those younger than 30 years, should be screened for chlamydia before any uterine instrumentation, using an appropriately sensitive technique. Alternatively, antibiotic prophylaxis, for example with doxycycline, may be considered. It is recommended that where chlamydial infection is discovered there should be a local mechanism whereby the disease can be notified and sexual partners treated. Collaboration with a genitourinary clinic is advisable.

MALE

The capacity of sperm to fertilise an egg depends on a complex series of biological events that includes transport to the site of fertilisation, sperm–egg recognition, the acrosome reaction and fusion of the sperm to the oocyte. The value of the postcoital test (PCT) in providing information about sperm function in the male is still disputed. A review of the literature would suggest that the test lacks validity for routine use. Nevertheless, if sexual dysfunction is suspected, or the male partner cannot or will not provide a semen sample for analysis, the PCT may have a place, even at an early stage in investigations. It is crucial that the test is done at the correct stage in the cycle; that is, at the time of maximal cervical mucus production before ovulation. Inappropriate timing of the test may provide misleading information and cause unnecessary concern. Ideally, mucus production should be assessed daily using an objective method. Occasionally, mucus production may be poor until the day of the beginning of the LH surge and this may indicate a functional problem within the cervix, an unusual situation even in cases where there has been previous cervical surgery. This need for precise timing leads to a sex-on-demand approach to investigation, which may produce additional strain and tension for an already overburdened couple, trying to cope with the stress of their infertility and their associated loss of self-esteem.

Other tests of sperm function, including computerised analysis of sperm movement characteristics, sperm cervical mucus penetration tests and DNA fragmentation, are not recommended for routine use, nor is testing for antisperm antibodies in semen. The place for such tests is discussed in Chapter 2.

Reaching a diagnosis

The management of people with infertility problems is largely dictated by the major diagnostic category into which they fit. Typical figures are shown in Table 1.5.

Table 1.5 Diagnostic categories and distribution of couples with primary and secondary infertility

Diagnostic category	Infertility	
	Primary (%)	Secondary (%)
Male factor	25	20
Disorders of ovulation	20	15
Tubal factor	15	40
Endometriosis	10	5
Unexplained	30	20

Diagnostic categories in most studies include male factors, disorders of ovulation, tubal factors, endometriosis and uterine factors related to infertility, and unexplained infertility. The distribution of causes, when analysed, is affected by whether the female has been pregnant in the past (that is, secondary infertility). This has an association with an increased risk of tubal factor infertility compared with those couples with primary infertility (that is, where there has not been a pregnancy in the past). The possibility that male factors may contribute to a couple's infertility should not be ignored even where the man has fathered a pregnancy in the past.

It should be borne in mind that more than one factor may contribute to a couple's infertility and each may require simultaneous management, for example ovulation induction for a woman who is not ovulating in combination with donor insemination. Decisions to initiate active treatment will be influenced by the age of the female partner, the duration of infertility and whether or not there has been a pregnancy in the past. Initiating intrusive and potentially harmful treatment should take account of natural expectations of pregnancy. In many instances, expectant management will be appropriate.

Prognosis

It is generally accepted that the three most important factors determining the chance of natural or assisted conception in the infertile are the age of the female partner, the duration of infertility and whether there has been a conception previously. Once a diagnosis is reached, any judgement on the prognosis for conception must take these issues into account. In addition, it is important when making a judgement about interventions to consider the potential hazards of treatment for the female partner as well as potential harm to offspring.

For male factor infertility, which accounts for up to 25% of cases, the impairment of fertility may be exaggerated if the female partner is in her advanced reproductive years. Some men with impaired fertility may not present to t he fertility clinic if the female partner is of above average fertility herself.

Ovulatory disorders, often associated with irregular menstruation, are associated with reduced chances of natural conception. Ovulation induction provides good chances of success if there are no other complicating factors such as tubal compromise or severe impairment in sperm quality. Significantly overweight women are less responsive to treatment. The outlook for women with ovarian failure is very pessimistic.

Tubal factor infertility, which accounts for up to 30% of cases, may have profound effects on the chances of natural conception, particularly if severe pelvic distortion is present.

Unexplained infertility accounts for around one-quarter of the couples seen in fertility clinics. Treatment-independent conceptions are a particular issue in this group of patients in our evaluation of the cost-effectiveness of interventions. In younger patients with short duration of infertility, expectant management will be appropriate; in older patients, this may not be the best option.

These issues will be discussed in much greater detail in other chapters in this book.

Conclusion

The preliminary assessment of egg and sperm availability, together with a determination that the gametes can meet, should provide a diagnosis for the majority of couples. In most cases, a prognosis, usually favourable, can be given to the couple. Appropriate therapeutic strategies can be instituted where required, with specialist involvement if necessary. The lines of communication within a regional framework should be set out clearly, with the involvement of GPs intimately linked to the process of assessment. Clinical protocols should be clearly set out so that unnecessary repetition of investigations is minimised. Clinics should be structured so that the same practitioner sees patients as far as possible and if subspecialist help is required this should be readily available. Information leaflets are a valuable adjunct to the smooth running of the clinic and suitably trained nursing staff should be an integral part of the service, providing a day-to-day focus for patient contact.

Such personnel can plan and coordinate treatment protocols on an individual basis and, linked to a sympathetic counselling service, will be able to best serve the considerable and complex needs of the infertile population entrusted to their care.

KEY POINTS

- A pragmatic definition of infertility is an inability to conceive after 1 year but occasionally specialist referral may be required in advance of this.
- One in six couples experience difficulty in conceiving at some point in their reproductive life.
- Education on maximising health for pregnancy and on awareness and prevention of infertility should be part of public health policy.
- Good liaison between the GP and specialist clinic-based services is essential.
- Assessment should be complete within 3–4 months and a prognosis given dependent on the diagnosis, female age, duration of infertility and history of previous pregnancy.
- In many cases, the prognosis will be favourable without intervention but those seeking advice will often require psychological support.

Further reading

National Collaborating Centre for Women's and Children's Health, National Institute for Health and Clinical Excellence (2013) *Fertility: Assessment and Treatment for People with Fertility Problems.* 2nd ed. London: Royal College of Obstetricians and Gynaecologists [http://guidance.nice.org.uk/CG156/Guidance].

Hamilton M (2009) Infertility. In: Mahmood T, Templeton A, Dhillon C, editors. *Models of Care in Women's Health*. London: RCOG Press. p. 24–34.

Evers JL (2002) Female subfertility. *Lancet* 360:151–9.

Bhattacharya S, Porter M, Amalraj E, Templeton A, Hamilton M, Lee AJ, et al. (2009) The epidemiology of infertility in the North East of Scotland. *Hum Reprod* 24:3096–107.

2 Male factor infertility

Introduction

The definition of male factor infertility is fraught with problems. At the simplest level, it only takes one sperm to fertilise one egg. However, ejaculated sperm have to find the cervix, traverse the cervical canal, swim through the uterine cavity, pick the correct fallopian tube and then reach its ampulla before finding the egg and fertilising it. Estimating a man's fertility is additionally complicated by the fact that there is a significant variation between sperm samples and, indeed, between the results obtained by different technicians analysing the same sample. Estimating a man's fertility is thus rather like putting 'betting odds' on his chances of becoming a father: the more healthy sperm there are the greater the chances of conception, but what is the lower limit at which a man has, in effect, no chance of fathering a child?

It is estimated that male factor problems are primarily responsible for up to 25% of cases of infertility and may be contributory in a further 20%. Assisted reproductive technology (ART) techniques such as intracytoplasmic sperm injection (ICSI) have revolutionised the treatment of infertility and allowed men with severe oligozoospermia, and many with azoospermia, to father their own children. Despite the success of such techniques, many of the underlying problems contributing to male infertility remain unidentified and unexplored.

Aetiology

The aetiology of male factor infertility is broadly divided into genetic and acquired causes. The genetic causes are proving particularly difficult to identify, although the azoospermia factor (AZF) region of the Y chromosome is certainly associated with some cases. The environmental causes are equally difficult to confirm, probably because any effect is relative rather than absolute and most relevant studies, certainly in humans, need to be observational rather than randomised. The much-vaunted reports of falling sperm counts are also dogged with controversy: are similar populations being assessed over the years and, indeed, are similar techniques of assessment being used? Any decline in semen parameters has yet to be linked with decreased fertility. However, at least in animals, the effect of increased environmental estrogenic compounds is of concern, though unproven. In humans, while a number of endocrine-disrupting compounds have been linked to the rising incidence of cryptorchidism and testicular cancer, this association is not yet proven either.

Most men presenting with infertility can thus not be given an explanation as to the cause of the problem, nor can an underlying pathology be identified. A study published by the World Health Organization (WHO) found no demonstrable cause in almost 50% of couples with male factor infertility. The distribution of diagnoses when male factor subfertility was encountered in the WHO study is shown in Table 2.1.

Table 2.1 Causes of male factor infertility

Cause	Incidence (%)
No demonstrable cause	48.8
Varicocele	12.6
Idiopathic oligozoospermia	11.2
Accessory gland infection	6.9
Idiopathic teratozoospermia	5.9
Idiopathic asthenozoospermia	3.9
Isolated seminal plasma abnormalities	3.5
Suspected immunological subfertility	3.0
Congenital abnormalities	1.7
Systemic diseases	1.4
Sexual inadequacy	1.3
Obstructive azoospermia	<1
Idiopathic necrozoospermia	<1
Ejaculatory inadequacy	<1
Hyperprolactinaemia	<1
Iatrogenic causes	<1
Karyotype abnormalities	<1
Partial obstruction to ejaculatory duct	<1
Retrograde ejaculation	<1
Immotile cilia syndrome	<1
Pituitary lesions	<1
Gonadotrophin deficiency	<1

Source: World Health Organization (1992) The influence of varicocele on parameters of fertility in a large group of men presenting to infertility clinics. *Fertil Steril* 57:1289–93.

TESTICULAR EMBRYOLOGY AND SPERM PRODUCTION

Testicular development is primarily controlled by the Y chromosome. The embryonic germ cells migrate to the genital ridge and populate the seminiferous tubules, which are formed from the Wolffian ducts. Sertoli cells develop directly from the embryonic genital ridge and secrete antimüllerian hormone (AMH), thereby inducing regression of the müllerian ducts, which would otherwise develop into the female pelvic organs. Leydig cells then appear, producing testosterone, which induces the development of the Wolffian duct structures via androgen receptors. Gradually, the maturing testes migrate down to the pelvis and through the inguinal canal into the scrotum. The development of the male genitalia is, therefore, dependent on testosterone, androgen receptors and 5α-reductase, which converts testosterone to dihydrotestosterone (DHT).

In adult life, each man has approximately 1 km of seminiferous tubules (Figure 2.1). On the outer aspect is the basement membrane that forms the blood–testis barrier and renders the interior of the tubule and its contents hidden from the normal immunological processes. The diploid germ cells lie on the basement membrane and the Sertoli cells extend from the basement membrane to the lumen of the tubule. These cells are the nursemaid cells that control the development of the diploid germ cell into the mature haploid sperm. Interspersed between the Sertoli cells are the Leydig cells that produce the androgens essential to normal testicular development and sperm production.

The process of germ cell maturation should be thought of as producing a machine to transfer paternal DNA to the egg and into the ooplasm. Thus, as the germ cell matures it becomes haploid and sheds almost all of its organelles and cytoplasmic fluid, making sperm one of the smallest cells known. The mitochondria

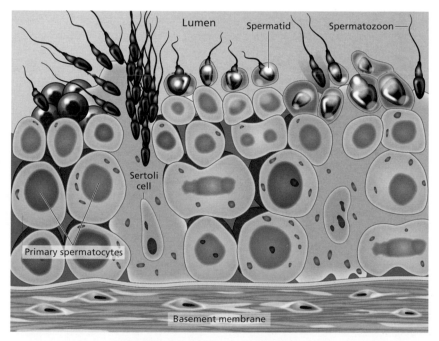

Figure 2.1 Schematic of sperm production

become ensheathed around the proximal ends of the tail fibrils, in the midpiece of the sperm, thus focusing their energy production where it is needed. The nuclear DNA becomes very tightly condensed and packaged and largely inactive. Finally, an acrosome is formed from the Golgi apparatus and lies in front of the nucleus. It contains hyaluronidase and acrosin, enzymes specifically designed to help the sperm penetrate the granulosa cell layers surrounding the oocyte.

In the broadest sense, follicle-stimulating hormone (FSH) controls sperm production and exerts its effects primarily on the Sertoli cells whilst luteinising hormone (LH) exerts its effects primarily on the Leydig cells and androgen production. Testosterone completes the negative feedback loop to the anterior pituitary for LH production whilst inhibin and activin, from the Sertoli cells, complete the negative feedback loop for FSH production.

VARICOCELE

A varicocele is a tortuous engorgement of the pampiniform venous plexus within the scrotum. This results in a swelling that is classically described as 'a bag of worms'. It has been linked to oligoasthenozoospermia but this is controversial as it is relatively common, occurring in 5–20% of the general population and 10–40% of infertile men. Most varicoceles are asymptomatic but some may cause a dragging discomfort on the affected side. They are usually found coincidentally during examination of the scrotum – more commonly on the left – and are classified as primary (idiopathic) or secondary. Primary varicoceles are more common and are thought to be due to an anatomical compression of the left renal vein between the aorta and the superior mesenteric artery (the nutcracker phenomenon) or to insufficiency of the valves in the left testicular vein. Either way, there is reflux of blood from the venocaval circulation down the left testicular vein to the pampiniform plexus of the testis.

Secondary varicoceles are rare and are due, for example, to obstruction of the left testicular vein by a growth (such as a hypernephroma) along the renal veins. Characteristically, these varicoceles do not decompress in the supine position.

WHO suggests that there is an inverse relationship between semen quality and the presence and severity of varicoceles, at least among the male partners of infertile couples. However, treatment of varicoceles by ligation of the spermatic vein or radiological embolisation is not clearly associated with either an improvement in semen parameters or pregnancy rates.

HYPOGONADOTROPHIC HYPOGONADISM

The rare condition of hypogonadotrophic hypogonadism may be caused by hypothalamic or pituitary failure and can be congenital or acquired. Patients usually present with clinical evidence of androgen deficiency at around the time of puberty. However, adult-onset (post-pubertal) hypogonadotrophic hypogonadism may be recognised in males presenting with infertility due, for example, to trauma, tumour, chronic inflammatory lesions or iron overload.

In congenital hypogonadotrophic hypogonadism, a complete absence of gonadotrophin-releasing hormone (GnRH) results in the absence of secondary sexual development and total testicular failure, with small, atrophic testes. However, males with a partial deficiency will have less profound manifestations of the disorder, with larger but still underdeveloped testes. Most of these patients will have anosmia or hyposmia (Kallmann syndrome). Low or undetectable levels of gonadotrophins (LH and FSH), which lead to lack of spermatogenesis and low testosterone levels, usually confirm the diagnosis.

COITAL DYSFUNCTION

Coital dysfunction is perhaps under-reported by many couples. Psychosexual dysfunction is more common than physiological coital dysfunction but both are uncommon causes of male infertility. It should be noted that the accompanying stress associated with investigations and treatment for infertility can induce this problem where it did not previously exist. A list of causes of coital dysfunction is given in Table 2.2.

The main physiological cause of impotence is hyperprolactinaemia, which accounts for 1–5% of cases. Endocrine disorders such as androgen deficiency and

Table 2.2 Aetiology of coital dysfunction

Problem	Can result from ...
Ejaculatory failure	• spinal cord injury • medical disorders: o multiple sclerosis o diabetes o chronic renal failure • bladder-neck surgery • retroperitoneal lymph node dissection
Erectile or ejaculatory problems	• depression • alcohol abuse • medication: o adrenergic blocking agents o antihypertensive agents o psychotrophic agents • psychosexual
Loss of libido and impotence	• hyperprolactinaemia due to: o pituitary adenomas o chronic renal failure o idiopathic o drug therapy
Retrograde ejaculation	• transurethral prostatectomy • retroperitoneal lymph node dissection • diabetic neuropathy due to: o injury to the lumbar sympathetic nerves o damage to the neck of the bladder

hypothyroidism can also lead to coital dysfunction but usually present with other clinical manifestations of the specific disorder.

Imaging of the hypothalamic–pituitary axis is mandatory in all patients with sexual dysfunction in the presence of elevated prolactin levels.

Retrograde ejaculation is the propulsion of seminal fluid from the posterior urethra into the bladder rather than along the urethra. The diagnosis is made by the absence of ejaculate (aspermia) and the presence of significant numbers of spermatozoa in a post-ejaculatory urine specimen. Retrograde ejaculation is not uncommon in men with diabetes and in those with multiple sclerosis or transection of the spinal cord. However, it can also occur secondary to benign hypertrophy of the prostate or to transurethral resection of the prostate. Drugs, especially selective serotonin reuptake inhibitors (SSRIs) can also temporarily induce the problem.

IMMUNOLOGICAL CAUSES

Antisperm antibodies, which may be present in serum or seminal plasma or be bound to sperm, have been associated with infertility but their significance is not clear – low levels are certainly unlikely to be of clinical relevance. Antisperm antibodies are usually immunoglobulin G (IgG) or A (IgA) and can be variously bound to the sperm head, midpiece and/or tail. Given that sperm are produced in an immunologically privileged site, the production of antibodies is presumably secondary to some traumatic event that resulted in a breach of the testis–blood barrier. Significant risk factors include vasectomy (and vasectomy reversal), infections such as epididymitis and orchitis, and direct trauma – for example, in sports injuries. However, in the majority of cases no such event can be identified.

Antibodies may reduce male fertility by literally weighing down the affected sperm and reducing their motility, causing sperm to clump together (agglutinate), or, by covering the head of the sperm, preventing them from binding effectively to the oocyte or impairing the release of their acrosomal enzymes.

GENITAL TRACT INFECTION

Acute clinical infections of the genital tract (orchitis, epididymitis, prostatovesiculitis or urethritis) typically present with pain and possibly fever. The initial consequence of such an infection is a decrease in semen quality but this is reversible with treatment. However, in the longer term, infection may result in complete obstruction of the epididymis or vas deferens and cause azoospermia. Gram-negative enterococci, chlamydia and gonococcus are the most commonly implicated organisms. In addition, acute bacterial infections of the genital tract or sexually transmitted infection (STIs) can lead to infection of the accessory glands resulting in permanent structural damage and scarring, with obstruction to the outflow tract. It is obvious that all genital infections should be treated with appropriate antibiotics as quickly as possible and after a full genitourinary evaluation by a sexual health specialist.

Symptomatic orchitis also occurs in around one-third of males over 11 years of age who are diagnosed with mumps. The prevalence of infertility after viral orchitis is unknown but impaired fertility occurs in bilateral orchitis owing to seminiferous tubular atrophy and impairment of spermatogenesis. Prepubertal orchitis is much less significant in terms of effects on future fertility than the post-pubertal version.

NON-INFECTIVE CAUSES OF GENITAL TRACT OBSTRUCTION

Non-infective obstruction is a rare cause of azoospermia and can be associated with the cystic fibrosis gene. Azoospermia may be present in men with none of the respiratory or gastrointestinal complications of the condition. In men with cystic fibrosis, the vas deferens will be found to be absent bilaterally on clinical examination. Overall, however, vasectomy, either intentional or accidental (at the time of other surgery such as hernia repair), is the most common cause of genital tract obstruction in men. The outcome of surgical correction is highly variable, depending, in large part, on the skill of the surgeon and the techniques used. However, a vasectomy of more than 10 years' standing is unlikely to be surgically correctable and the combination of testicular biopsy and ICSI represents the greatest chance of pregnancy. It should be noted that the incidence of antisperm antibodies in successful vasectomy reversal cases is at least 50%.

TESTICULAR MALDESCENT AND TESTICULAR DYSGENESIS SYNDROME

It is now accepted that the trilogy of testicular maldescent, oligoasthenoteratozoospermia and testicular cancer are inextricably linked. Anyone with one of these conditions is at an increased risk for the other two. Failure of the hypothalamic–pituitary–gonadal axis may also rarely be associated with failure of testicular descent. While maldescent of the testes is present in 3–6% of males at term birth, in the majority of these it resolves spontaneously by the age of 2 years, giving an overall incidence of around 1%. It is now accepted that an abnormal position of the testis should be corrected by the end of the first year of life.

Germ cell degeneration and dysplasia may be a direct result of maldescent or may be present as part of testicular dysgenesis syndrome. Early surgical correction is clearly associated with improved spermatogenesis, decreased risk of testicular cancer and beneficial psychological effects but these advantages cannot be guaranteed.

CHROMOSOMAL ABNORMALITIES

The most common chromosomal disorder affecting spermatogenesis is Klinefelter syndrome (47,XXY). Fifteen percent of azoospermic men and 4% of oligozoospermic men have an abnormal karyotype. An incidence of 2.2% for chromosomal abnormalities was detected in over 2000 men attending a male subfertility clinic over a 10-year period. These abnormalities also included reciprocal

X or Y autosomal translocations, and XYY and XX males. Males with azoospermia or severe oligozoospermia (less than 5 M/ml) should have a karyotype performed. In addition, an AZF test for Y chromosome deletions in this region is advisable for those with azoospermia as the absence of various AZF sub-types is associated with varying prognoses in terms of the likelihood of finding sperm at testicular biopsy.

CHEMOTHERAPY, RADIOTHERAPY AND TOXINS

Treatment with certain drugs or exposure to radiation or chemicals can affect actively dividing germ cells causing defective spermatogenesis (Table 2.3), and this may be temporary or permanent. Anabolic steroids, used typically by body builders, also interfere with feedback to the pituitary, causing a reduction in gonadotrophin secretion and a decrease in, if not a total absence of, sperm production. The associated testicular atrophy is reversible.

Table 2.3   Therapeutic drugs interfering with male fertility

Drug	Note
Cancer chemotherapy	Effects are variable; all men undergoing such treatment should be offered long-term sperm storage
Antibiotics	Some evidence of damage in animal studies but all effects are reversible on cessation of treatment
Hormone treatment	Androgens and anti-androgens can suppress sperm production
Cimetidine	May compete with androgens at receptor level; may raise prolactin levels
Spironolactone	Has some anti-androgenic effects
Aminosalicylates	Were thought to decrease sperm counts but evidence is poor and any effect is likely to be minimal

Chemotherapeutic drugs used for the treatment of various malignancies can also have a deleterious effect on fertility and many patients will become azoospermic within 8 weeks of commencing treatment. Alkylating agents may cause irreversible damage.

Radiotherapy to the testes destroys germ cells with an irreversible arrest of spermatogenesis. Almost invariably, this results in permanent sterility.

Toxins in the workplace and environment may also cause damage to the germ cells. A well-documented example is the chemical dibromochloropropane (DBCP), which, in one report, caused azoospermia in 14 of 25 exposed males. It is thus always good practice to take a detailed work history from men with abnormal semen parameters.

IDIOPATHIC MALE INFERTILITY

Even after meticulous evaluation, up to 50% of those with male factor subfertility have no demonstrable cause for their condition. A diagnosis of idiopathic infertility can only be made after all other causes of infertility have been excluded. Semen analysis may show varying degrees of abnormality, which may be associated with elevated serum FSH, indicating failure of spermatogenesis. It is quite possible that a significant percentage of these cases are associated with so far unelucidated genetic aberrations.

AETIOLOGY OF MALE FACTOR INFERTILITY: KEY POINTS

- Varicoceles are possibly associated with impaired testicular function and infertility.
- Psychosexual dysfunction as a primary cause of male infertility is uncommon.
- Imaging of the hypothalamic–pituitary axis is mandatory in all patients with impotence and elevated prolactin levels.
- At least 50% of males have clinically significant antisperm antibodies after vasectomy and this is of clinical importance if reversal is required.
- The most common cause of genital tract obstruction is iatrogenic following vasectomy.
- Maldescent of the testes occurs in 3–6% of males at birth and should be corrected by the end of the first year of life.
- Males with azoospermia or severe oligozoospermia (less than 5 M/ml) should have a karyotype performed.
- Up to 50% of those with male factor subfertility have no demonstrable cause.

Clinical management

Both partners must always be involved in the investigation and management of infertility. However, the relevance of any male factor must be judged against other factors, such as female age, the duration of infertility and any history of previous conceptions, when managing a couple with suboptimal semen parameters.

HISTORY AND EXAMINATION

It is all too common to gloss over the male history. However, obtaining a detailed history is mandatory to exclude exposure to spermato-toxins and spermato-toxic events as well as to determine the general health and wellbeing of the male.

It is arguable that it is only necessary to examine the male partner when there is an abnormality of the semen parameters. This is described in Chapter 1.

Investigations

SEMEN ANALYSIS

Semen analysis is one of the fundamental investigations of the infertile couple irrespective of whether the man has previously fathered children or not (see Chapter 1). It should be performed according to recognised WHO methodology. Laboratories undertaking this test should have a mechanism for internal quality control as well as access to an external quality control scheme. If the first specimen shows an abnormality, it is good practice to repeat the semen sample after a gap of at least 1 month. If the semen analysis is abnormal or there is cause for concern in the history or on clinical examination, further investigation of the male partner should be undertaken in a secondary or tertiary centre (see Chapter 1, Table 1.3 for reference values).

There has been an increased interest in sperm DNA tests in the last decade. However, these tests are hampered by high inter- and intra-assay variability and they are simply an assessment of the overall amount of damage in the sperm DNA. They do not, for example, allow the selection of sperm with low DNA damage as all of the tests available involve destroying the sperm as part of the analysis. It is questionable whether they have any useful clinical role at present.

ENDOCRINE TESTS

Endocrine tests include:

- serum FSH
- serum testosterone
- prolactin.

Serum FSH

Serum FSH should be measured in a male partner with azoospermia or severe oligozoospermia (sperm density less than 5 M/ml). It is particularly useful in differentiating between non-obstructive and obstructive azoospermia, where there is normal spermatogenesis. In non-obstructive cases there is failure of spermatogenesis and the FSH values will be significantly elevated.

FSH estimation also gives prognostic information in men prior to testicular biopsy if ICSI is being considered, although a high value does not totally exclude the possibility of sperm recovery. Nevertheless, a value over 15 iu/l is a bad prognostic sign.

Serum testosterone

Serum testosterone is only indicated if hypogonadism is suspected. Males with hypogonadism of hypothalamic or pituitary origin will have low FSH, LH and testosterone levels.

Prolactin

Virtually all men with hyperprolactinaemia have sexual dysfunction. It is mandatory to check for elevated prolactin levels in men complaining of loss of libido and particularly impotence. Imaging of the hypothalamic–pituitary axis is indicated in males with high prolactin levels to detect tumours such as prolactinoma, craniopharyngioma or tumours compressing the pituitary stalk.

It should be borne in mind that elevated prolactin levels might also occur in men on medication such as tranquillisers and sulpiride.

MICROBIOLOGICAL ASSESSMENT OF SEMEN

The biological significance of the presence of white blood cells in semen and asymptomatic subclinical infection is unclear. In addition, many organisms are urethral contaminants and of very doubtful clinical significance. Semen culture should be performed in males with microscopic evidence of infection (the presence of white cells in the semen, or organisms) as well as those with symptoms of orchitis, epididymitis or prostatitis. Male partners of women with acute tubal disease should also be screened.

IMAGING OF THE GENITAL TRACT

Diagnostic tests of varicocele

Varicocele can be diagnosed by thermography, ultrasound with Doppler blood flow (higher false-positive rate), radionuclide angiography (higher false-negative rate) or retrograde venography. The last is the gold standard test, although it is invasive and usually unnecessary as it is likely that only large varicoceles are of clinical significance.

Scrotal ultrasound scan

Scrotal ultrasound is not performed routinely but should be undertaken if testicular tumours are suspected. In addition, an ultrasound may be helpful in detecting hydroceles and epididymal cysts and may be better than clinical examination.

Vasography

Vasography is performed in men with obstruction to the vas deferens and usually takes place in theatre before surgery in order to determine the level of obstruction.

TESTICULAR BIOPSY

Testicular biopsy was initially used as a diagnostic tool to differentiate between obstructive and non-obstructive azoospermia but this has now largely been replaced by serum FSH measurements. Testicular biopsy should be carried out only in tertiary centres where there are trained staff and facilities for sperm recovery and cryopreservation. In addition, a pathologist experienced in assessing testicular histology is an essential member of the team.

Sperm recovered during biopsy can be used for ICSI, giving azoospermic men the opportunity to father their own genetic offspring. Cryopreservation facilities should be available since sperm recovered might not be used for ICSI immediately. Additionally, should sperm extraction not be carried out at the same time as the biopsy, this may affect future attempts at sperm recovery owing to the possibility of trauma and devascularisation, of fibrosis or of an autoimmune response.

While open testicular biopsies are still performed, the majority of cases can be easily dealt with using a needle biopsy technique under local anaesthetic.

GENETIC STUDIES

Karyotyping/DNA analysis for Y chromosome microdeletions

Males with azoospermia or severe oligozoospermia should have a karyotype analysis. In addition, in cases of azoospermia, AZF deletions should be looked for.

Cystic fibrosis screen

Congenital bilateral absence of the vas deferens (CBAVD) is, in the majority of patients, related to defects in the cystic fibrosis transmembrane conductance regulator (*CFTR*) gene. CBAVD is frequently associated with heterozygosity for the common cystic fibrosis gene mutation ΔF508. A mutation analysis should be performed in males with CBAVD and, if positive, the female partner should be screened for cystic fibrosis as any resulting children will have an increased risk of being born with this condition and/or CBAVD.

Antisperm antibodies

Testing for antisperm antibodies should be routinely offered in tertiary centres. While there is no evidence of effective treatment to improve fertility, their presence, especially in high percentages, would direct the couple towards assisted reproduction rather than other less invasive options for otherwise unexplained infertility such as intrauterine insemination (IUI).

Postcoital test

This test has been abandoned in many centres. Both the inter- and intra-assay coefficients of variation are high and a couple might be directed towards more invasive treatments such as in vitro fertilisation (IVF) unnecessarily early.

INVESTIGATIONS: KEY POINTS

- Female age, duration of infertility and history of previous pregnancy should be taken into account when interpreting the semen analysis for the individual couple.
- Clinical examination of the male is important and should always be undertaken where there is a significant male factor problem on semen analysis.
- Should semen analysis or clinical examination reveal abnormalities, further management should be undertaken in specialised centres.
- Serum FSH has virtually replaced testicular biopsy in differentiating between obstructive azoospermia and non-obstructive azoospermia but the latter remains a particularly useful method for obtaining sperm for storage for subsequent attempts at assisted reproduction.
- The postcoital test is a poor predictor of fertility and has been largely abandoned as part of the infertility 'work-up'.

Treatment

GENERAL MANAGEMENT

There is an increasing amount of evidence that advancing age has a detrimental effect on male fertility. Alcohol consumption within the Department of Health's recommendations is unlikely to affect fertility; however, excessive alcohol intake is detrimental to semen quality. Men who smoke should be advised to stop although the evidence of any improvement on standard semen analysis parameters is poor. There is, however, evidence of increased sperm DNA damage in heavy smokers. The actual impact of this on male fertility remains, however, uncertain.

The use of so-called recreational drugs has also been linked to a decrease in male fertility but the quality of the evidence is, again, poor. However, as with smoking, there is evidence of increased sperm DNA damage in men who use cannabis regularly. It is obvious that any anabolic steroid use must be stopped.

A number of myths have developed around a link between tight underwear, hot baths, mobile phones, laptop computers etc. and a decrease in male fertility. The evidence for these associations is at best very tenuous and physiologically makes little sense: the testes have a rich blood supply, one of the actions of which is to maintain core testicular temperature. It is hard to see that the use of tight underwear would make any significant difference to this.

MANAGEMENT OF VARICOCELE

In the light of current evidence, there is no justification for treating men with a clinically detectable varicocele but a normal sperm count. This does not appear to improve pregnancy rates. The evidence for treating oligozoospermic men is uncertain and benefit is far from clear. However, if the varicocele is symptomatic, it should be treated.

The surgical approach involves ligation of the spermatic vein above the inguinal ligament at the internal inguinal ring. Only occasionally is a local excision indicated, for example in cases where ligation leaves a group of tortuous varicosities. Alternatively, and increasingly commonly, testicular vein embolisation is employed under radiological guidance.

MANAGEMENT OF GONADOTROPHIN DEFICIENCY

Hypogonadotrophic hypogonadism is one of the few conditions associated with male factor infertility that can be treated successfully with complete restoration of steroidogenesis and spermatogenesis (Table 2.4). Treatment is usually with FSH and human chorionic gonadotrophin (hCG) injections and results in effective spermatogenesis in 70–90% of men. It typically takes 3–6 months to achieve normal semen parameters. Testosterone replacement, for symptomatic hypogonadotrophic hypogonadism, will, of course, not result in the return of spermatogenesis.

Table 2.4 Summary of management of gonadotrophin deficiency

Treatment	Deficiency	Action	Administered as
hCG (source of LH activity)	Acquired HH	Stimulates Leydig cells to produce testosterone	Intramuscular injection 3 times per week
hCG + hMG (source of FSH)	Acquired/prepubertal HH	As above and causes maturation and proliferation of the germinal cells; stimulates spermatogenesis	Intramuscular injection 3 times per week
hCG + HP-FSH (better tolerated)	Acquired/prepubertal HH	Effective in stimulating spermatogenesis and steroidogenesis	Self-administered subcutaneously over months or years to achieve maximum testicular size and spermatogenesis
Pulsatile GnRH therapy	HH of hypothalamic origin	Stimulation of the pituitary and testis; stimulates spermatogenesis	Battery-driven portable infusion pump; administers set dose subcutaneously (worn continuously for about 1 year)
Dopamine agonists (bromocriptine)	HH due to prolactinomas (causing hyperprolactinaemia)	Normalises serum prolactin levels, LH secretion begins, testosterone levels normalise, restoration of potency and fertility	5–10 mg/day in divided doses

FSH = follicle-stimulating hormone; GnRH = gonadotrophin-releasing hormone; hCG = human chorionic gonadotrophin; hMG = human menopausal gonadotrophin; HH = hypogonadotrophic hypogonadism; HP-FSH = highly purified FSH; LH = luteinising hormone

MANAGEMENT OF EJACULATORY PROBLEMS

Counselling forms an important part of the management of couples with impotence secondary to psychosexual causes. The pathway for sexual arousal and stimulation leading to erection is the production of cyclic guanosine monophosphate (cGMP) in the corpus cavernosum, which relaxes the smooth muscle and causes blood to fill the corpora. The phosphodiesterase type 5 inhibitor drugs, such as sildenafil, specifically inhibit the isoenzyme cGMP-specific phosphodiesterase type 5, which is responsible for the breakdown of cGMP in the corpus cavernosum. This results in a good erectile response in many men. Although orgasmic function, satisfaction with intercourse and overall sexual function are improved, these drugs have no effect on sex drive. In addition, there is some laboratory-based evidence that they may be detrimental to sperm function and quality.

If drugs fail, alternatives include external vibratory massage, direct aspiration of sperm from the epididymis or testes, and electroejaculation. All methods tend to produce poor-quality sperm samples and most commonly they are only suitable for ICSI although with electroejaculation the sample may be suitable for IUI or IVF.

For retrograde ejaculation, the use of various drugs, including tricyclic antidepressants, antihistamines and nasal decongestants such as ephedrine and phenylephrine, has been reported. They clearly cannot work where the bladder sphincter is damaged but there is anecdotal evidence that these medical treatments are useful in some cases. They probably work by stimulating peristalsis in the vas deferens and by closing the bladder neck. Realistically, though, the most practical way to obtain sperm is from a urine sample taken immediately after masturbation. Some authorities recommend alkalinising the urine before the procedure, for example by the oral consumption of dissolved baking soda. This is probably unnecessary if the urine sample is going to be collected immediately after ejaculation and spun down within a few minutes.

IMMUNOLOGICAL INFERTILITY MANAGEMENT

Immunological male factor infertility refers to the presence of antisperm antibodies in the seminal fluid or bound to sperm. There was a time when high doses of corticosteroids were employed to suppress antisperm antibody levels but this practice has now largely been abandoned. There is no convincing evidence that it works and the adverse effects of the steroids range from dyspepsia, facial flushing, bloating, irritability, skin rashes and cushingoid appearance to the, albeit rare, serious complication of bilateral aseptic necrosis of the hip. It is current practice now to refer patients with high levels of IgA or IgG antibodies directly for ICSI.

MANAGEMENT OF GENITAL TRACT OBSTRUCTION

Reported success rates for vasectomy reversal vary from 17% to 82%. Factors influencing success rates include:

- the type of vasectomy
- the surgical technique employed (macro- or microsurgery) and the skill of the surgeon
- the presence of antisperm antibodies and, perhaps most importantly, the time since the vasectomy was performed.

Vasectomy reversal has some advantages over ICSI including the possibility of further spontaneous pregnancies without further intervention, conception following normal intercourse and the avoidance of the complications of assisted reproduction such as ovarian hyperstimulation syndrome (OHSS) and a highly significantly reduced chance of multiple pregnancy.

Where the obstruction is not iatrogenic, reconstructive surgical treatment should only be undertaken by trained surgeons with microsurgical skills in specialist centres with facilities for microsurgery, sperm retrieval and cryostorage. Increasingly, though, the first line of management for these cases is sperm retrieval by testicular biopsy followed by ICSI.

EMPIRICAL MEDICAL TREATMENTS

Gonadotrophins

FSH, hCG and human menopausal gonadotrophin (hMG) are successfully used in males with hypogonadotrophic hypogonadism and this has led to their use in idiopathic male infertility. However, there is no evidence to commend gonadotrophin treatment for idiopathic male infertility.

GnRH

GnRH has been used in males with idiopathic subnormal semen parameters but it has not been shown to improve semen parameters.

Androgens

Testosterone is required for normal spermatogenesis. This led to the use of androgens (such as mesterolone) in idiopathic male infertility but there is no evidence to support the effectiveness of this treatment. Testosterone exerts a negative feedback effect on the pituitary–gonadal axis, suppressing FSH and LH secretion and thereby adversely affecting spermatogenesis. Oral doses of testosterone required to achieve serum levels equivalent to intratesticular levels can cause hepatotoxicity. This therapeutic approach should be avoided.

Bromocriptine

Bromocriptine has been shown to be beneficial in men with hyperprolactinaemia, with or without hypogonadotrophic hypogonadism. In normo-gonadotrophic males it does not improve semen parameters or fertility.

Anti-estrogens

Clomifene or tamoxifen have been used for idiopathic male infertility. Many observational studies have shown apparent improvements in sperm concentration and/or motility as well as pregnancy rates. However, a review of randomised studies provided no proof of effectiveness of anti-estrogens and their use has, more recently, been abandoned in these circumstances in mainstream medicine.

Kallikrein

Kallikrein is a glycoprotein that causes release of kinins from kininogens. Although the mechanism of action of kallikrein is unclear, it has been suggested that a local increase in kinins at the testicular level influences spermatogenesis. In vitro studies have shown that kallikrein assists sperm motility and improves cervical mucus penetration. Following these observations, kallikrein was used in the treatment of idiopathic male infertility. However, recent randomised controlled studies have not shown any demonstrable benefits and, again, the drug should not be used.

Antioxidants

Antioxidants such as glutathione, vitamin E and vitamin C may improve semen parameters. Although there is some evidence of improved semen parameters and fertility, the use of antioxidants cannot, at present, be recommended as a useful therapeutic approach.

Mast-cell blockers

As with most other empirical drug treatments for male infertility, the use of mast-cell blockers to improve semen parameters has been dogged by small studies and, in many cases, very poor study design. There is no convincing evidence that these drugs have a useful clinical role in the management of oligoasthenoteratozoospermia.

ASSISTED REPRODUCTION

Self-insemination

Occasionally the situation arises where a man is able to ejaculate a semen sample by masturbation but cannot ejaculate during penetrative sexual intercourse. Here, it is entirely reasonable that the couple should be instructed in self-insemination. At the time of ovulation, the man produces his sample into a specimen cup and then, using a mixing needle, the sample is drawn into a syringe. The mixing needle is inserted high into the vagina and the sample deposited there. In the absence of other fertility pathologies, the pregnancy rates are excellent.

Superovulation and IUI

Superovulation and IUI (SIUI) appears to improve the relative odds of pregnancy in the presence of moderate abnormalities of the semen parameters. However, the actual pregnancy rates per cycle are low (4–6%). Therefore, there is a strong argument for bypassing SIUI and proceeding straight to ICSI.

ICSI

ICSI has become the gold standard treatment for male factor infertility. Even where the man has obstructive azoospermia, sperm may be obtained by testicular biopsy under local anaesthesia and used in this process. Pregnancy rates are comparable to those of standard IVF (Chapter 9).

Donor sperm insemination

The use of fresh normal donor sperm produces pregnancy rates entirely comparable to those of fertile couples. However, as sperm donation is an anonymous process, only quarantined sperm can be legally used in many countries, including the UK. Typically, a sperm donor is screened for a variety of infections including hepatitis, HIV and cytomegalovirus. If negative, he produces the sample and it is immediately placed in storage in liquid nitrogen. Six months after storage, the donor is rescreened and, if he remains negative for the various infections, the sample is released for clinical use. The problem lies in the fact that the freeze–thaw process compromises the motility of the sperm very significantly. Therefore, the pregnancy rates with both intracervical insemination and IUI are poor.

Given the national shortage of donor sperm, it is arguable that a couple requiring donor sperm should proceed straight to IVF, where pregnancy rates in excess of 30% can be obtained compared with rates of 5–10% in donor sperm insemination.

TREATMENT: KEY POINTS

- The significance of a varicocele in male factor infertility is controversial and corrective treatment is unlikely to be beneficial in terms of fertility.
- Gonadotrophins for hypogonadotrophic hypogonadism and bromocriptine for hyperprolactinaemia are effective treatments.
- The efficacy of medical treatment of retrograde ejaculation is disputable.
- Systemic steroids cannot be recommended for immunological infertility.
- Vasectomy reversal should be considered the first line of treatment in men requesting reversal of sterilisation where the vasectomy is relatively recent (typically of less than 10 years' standing).
- In male factor infertility, ICSI is the most effective treatment but it does expose the female to the complications of assisted reproduction and does not cure the underlying male problem.

Summary

Male factors are implicated in as many as 25% of couples with infertility. A systematic approach to evaluation using the principles of careful history taking, clinical examination and appropriate investigation should lead to timely assessment of prognosis and, in some cases, targeted intervention. Empirical medical treatment is now considered to be inappropriate. If the expectation of natural conception is low then the use of assisted reproductive technology (ART) is most often recommended. The risks of ART to patients and the welfare of potential offspring need to be factored in to clinical decision making.

Further reading

National Collaborating Centre for Women's and Children's Health, National Institute for Health and Clinical Excellence (2013) *Fertility: Assessment and Treatment for People with Fertility Problems.* 2nd ed. London: Royal College of Obstetricians and Gynaecologists [http://guidance.nice.org.uk/CG156/Guidance].

World Health Organization (1992) The influence of varicocele on parameters of fertility in a large group of men presenting to infertility clinics. *Fertil Steril* 57:1289–93.

World Health Organization (2010) *WHO Laboratory Manual for the Examination and Processing of Human Semen.* 5th ed. Geneva: WHO [http://whqlibdoc.who.int/publications/2010/9789241547789_eng.pdf].

3 Ovulatory disorders

Ovulatory dysfunction is a major contributory factor in 15–20% of couples presenting with infertility.

Physiology of ovulation

Menarche, at an average age of 13–14 years, reflects the commencement of ovulatory cycles resulting from the maturation of the hypothalamic–pituitary–ovarian axis. The normal female menstrual cycle comprises the processes of follicular development, ovulation, hormone production and response, and endometrial functional response over the course of a typical 28 days.

HYPOTHALAMIC FUNCTION

The hypothalamus secretes gonadotrophin-releasing hormone (GnRH) in a pulsatile fashion. Pulsatility commences before puberty and is responsible for the onset and continuation of gonadotrophin production by the pituitary gland. The production and release of these hormones is, however, modulated by feedback via the ovarian hormones estrogen and progesterone acting at the level of the pituitary and hypothalamus. GnRH secretion continues throughout the reproductive lifetime although its pulsatility and concentration changes over time.

PITUITARY AND OVARIAN FUNCTION

The gonadotrophins follicle-stimulating hormone (FSH) and luteinising hormone (LH) are secreted by the anterior pituitary gland. FSH is primarily responsible for follicular development in the ovary from the preantral follicle stage to maturity. The mechanism of negative feedback by ovarian estrogen and inhibin B derived from the cohort of available antral follicles modifies FSH production, thereby contributing to the limited maturation of just one or two follicles ultimately. Increasing estrogen production from the ovary results in the midcycle surge of LH by virtue of positive feedback at the level of the anterior pituitary. This surge stimulates ovulation of the mature follicle(s) as well as the resumption of the final meiotic division of the oocyte in preparation for fertilisation. The follicle then undergoes luteinisation and becomes known as the corpus luteum, which continues to produce estrogen as well as progesterone. After about a week (typically around day 21 of a 28-day cycle) in the absence of pregnancy, the corpus luteum begins to involute with reduced secretory function, finally resolving into the corpus albicans, essentially an inactive 'scar' in the ovarian cortex. Estrogen and progesterone concentrations return to a basal level.

THE MENSTRUAL OR ENDOMETRIAL CYCLE

In the first half of the menstrual cycle, follicular growth results in a rise of estrogen concentration, which promotes proliferation of the endometrium. This thickened endometrium is converted to secretory tissue under the influence of progesterone following ovulation. This prepares the endometrium for implantation by making it receptive to the conceptus. Menstruation typically follows 14 days after ovulation in a nonpregnant cycle because the decline in ovarian hormones from the involuting corpus luteum will no longer support it. The endometrium is then shed.

A normal menstrual cycle, however, is considered to last anything from 24 to 35 days, with ovulation usually occurring 14 days before the subsequent period.

OVARIAN RESERVE

The ovary contains a complement of oocytes available for maturation and ovulation. These oocytes were laid down in the ovary at the time of embryogenesis such that there is a finite number to last the woman's reproductive lifetime. The majority of oocytes are lost before birth. Most of the remaining oocytes are then lost before puberty and at the onset of ovulatory cycles some 500 000 oocytes remain. Menopause occurs when there are few remaining oocytes and non-functioning or poorly functioning follicles in the ovaries that are then unable to maintain an ovulatory response. There is a decline in both the number of follicles within the ovary as it ages (ovarian reserve) and the quality of the oocytes over time. A low ovarian reserve is characterised by a high basal (menstrual) FSH concentration (usually tested on days 2–4 of menses), a low antral follicle count (AFC) at early proliferative phase ultrasound scan or a low concentration of antimüllerian hormone (AMH). Ovulation induction treatments are less likely to be successful in women with low ovarian reserves.

Ovulatory dysfunction

Ovulatory dysfunction accounts for around 30% of female fertility problems. Abnormalities in ovulation can arise from a number of points in the hypothalamic–pituitary–ovarian axis. Abnormalities of hypothalamic pulsatile secretion of GnRH result in downstream lack of effectors and non-functioning ovaries. Similarly, pituitary dysfunction leads to non-stimulation of ovaries and failure of follicular development and ovulation. A primary problem of ovarian function, either congenital or acquired, may prevent normal ovulatory function.

Ovulatory dysfunction may result from a lack of available oocytes or of follicles. It may also result from a lack of sensitivity of the ovary to the stimulating hormones, for example where there are gonadotrophin receptor abnormalities;

this is rarely determined and, in practical terms, it may be indistinguishable from ovarian failure due to low follicle numbers. Finally, ovarian dysfunction may occur because of follicular developmental arrest, as is apparent in polycystic ovary syndrome (PCOS). PCOS is the most common cause of anovulatory infertility, with a population prevalence of 6–7%.

Clinical presentation of ovulatory dysfunction

CLINICAL FEATURES SUGGESTIVE OF OVULATION

An ovulating woman may be aware of a number of associated symptoms, with menstruation being the most obvious one. At the time of ovulation, some women are aware of it as a unilateral, short-lived and sharp pain, which is known as mittelschmerz (German for 'middle pain'). The influence of estrogen on the cervix results in the alteration of the normal creamy vaginal discharge to a watery clear consistency, which women may notice forms long strings on wiping, a quality known as spinnbarkeit (German for 'spinnability'). This is the time when women are most fertile – around ovulation and when cervical mucus is altered to allow sperm penetration. In the second half of the cycle, women may experience breast tenderness and other premenstrual symptoms, which resolve as menstruation commences.

SYMPTOMS OF OVULATORY DISORDERS

The absence of ovulation will result in the absence of the above ovulatory symptoms. Women who fail to ovulate will generally be rendered amenorrhoeic. Vaginal bleeding, if it occurs, may be considered to be dysfunctional and is likely to lack any clear pattern or predictability. Together with a lack of menses, there will be no mittelschmerz, spinnbarkeit or associated premenstrual symptoms.

Other symptoms may also occur as a result of anovulation. With absent follicular development, estrogen concentrations will remain basal and women may experience symptoms in relation to this. The exception is a diagnosis of PCOS, where there is a tonic secretion of estrogen above basal levels. This condition is discussed separately. A congenital or prepubertal aetiology will lead to the absence of, or incomplete, pubertal development, resulting in short stature, failure to develop secondary sexual characteristics, absent or immature pubic and axillary hair growth, and absent breast development. Symptoms of estrogen deficiency equivalent to the climacteric symptoms of vaginal dryness, reduced libido and other non-specific changes may also be experienced. A post-pubertal woman who has had prior ovarian activity may also experience hot flushes denoting estrogen withdrawal.

Ovulatory disorders

While there are common features in many cases, ovulatory problems are best considered by cause or level of lesion in the hypothalamic–pituitary–ovarian axis. The World Health Organization (WHO) classification is described in Table 3.1.

Table 3.1 WHO classification of ovulatory disorders

WHO classification	Description	Findings	Aetiology
Group 1	Hypogonadotrophic hypogonadism	Estradiol low FSH low LH low	Anorexia Extreme exercise Kallmann syndrome Sheehan syndrome Hyperprolactinaemia
Group 2		Estradiol normal FSH normal LH normal	PCOS
Group 3	Hypergonadotrophic hypogonadism	Estradiol low FSH high LH high	Turner syndrome Gonadal dysgenesis Fragile X syndrome Primary ovarian insufficiency Natural menopause

FSH = follicle-stimulating hormone; LH = luteinising hormone; PCOS = polycystic ovary syndrome
Source: Rowe PJ, Comhaire FH, Hargreave TB, Mellows HJ (1993) *WHO Manual for the Standardized Investigation and Diagnosis of the Infertile Couple*. Cambridge: Cambridge University Press

HYPOTHALAMIC–PITUITARY OVULATORY DISORDERS

Hypothalamic disorders may occur for many reasons but influences from higher centres in the brain are the most common aetiology for hypothalamic anovulation. Women who are stressed or underweight may become amenorrhoeic as a result. Women with a body mass index (BMI) below 18–19 kg/m^2 are at risk of hypothalamic anovulation and its consequences but this is particularly notable in the extreme situation of pathological eating disorders such as anorexia nervosa, where hypoestrogenaemia simply compounds the nutritional problems. Women such as ballerinas and world-class athletes who undertake high levels of exercise are often also rendered amenorrhoeic.

Hypothalamic–pituitary dysfunction leads to lack of stimulation of the ovarian cycle by lack of pituitary hormones. This may be an isolated problem, such as Kallmann syndrome associated with anosmia, which is a congenital gonadotrophin deficiency usually presenting as failure to enter puberty. Alternatively, global hypopituitarism may occur secondary to tumour growth and the destructive sequelae of both the tumour and its treatment (surgery and radiotherapy), or secondary to trauma, as in Sheehan syndrome where catastrophic hypovolaemic hypotension leads to secondary pituitary infarction and subsequent pan-hypopituitarism.

Pituitary abnormalities also include hyperprolactinaemia. Prolactin, normally secreted during breastfeeding, suppresses gonadotrophin secretion by action on the hypothalamus and may also directly inhibit FSH action at the follicular level. Prolactinomas, often microtumours in women, can present as secondary amenorrhoea or galactorrhoea, or both. Raised prolactin may also occur in association with macroadenomas of the pituitary and is also an effect of some antipsychotic medications such as phenothiazines.

PRIMARY OVARIAN INSUFFICIENCY

Primary ovarian insufficiency exists when the failure to ovulate results from an ovarian problem. There are two potential ovarian causes of ovarian insufficiency: one is that there are no longer eggs to be ovulated, the other that the ovary does not respond to FSH stimulation. Amenorrhoea results and endogenous gonadotrophin secretion increases significantly as the pituitary suppressive feedback is lost.

Congenital absence of follicles, or early follicular loss, results in poorly functioning or non-functioning ovaries, which, if they contain no oocytes from birth, may appear as fibrous 'streaks' at the pelvic brim. Turner syndrome (45,XO) is the most common cause of congenital streak ovaries. Any form of gonadal dysgenesis, however, may result in an adolescent girl failing to enter puberty and failing to initiate menstrual cycles. This includes testicular dysgenesis where a 46,XY karyotype is detected in a girl presenting in this way. As gonads are at risk of developing dysgerminoma, gonadectomy is recommended in this case.

Women with Turner mosaicism and fragile X syndrome, who have a low complement of oocytes, may go through puberty but experience an early menopause.

Primary ovarian insufficiency occurring after normal puberty is often idiopathic but may be associated with autoimmunity together with other autoimmune disorders, such as Addison's disease. Failure of the ovary to respond to FSH may also be iatrogenic from surgical intervention involving loss of normal ovary tissue, or following cancer treatments such as surgery, chemotherapy (particularly alkylating agents) and radiotherapy (pelvic or total body irradiation). Other causes include inherited metabolic disorders such as galactosaemia, which is associated with ovarian failure in adolescence. This disorder appears to lead to more rapid destruction of oocytes within the ovaries and to early deficiency.

A failure of ovarian response to stimulation despite the presence of primordial follicles and oocytes is rare but may result from FSH receptor (FSHR) abnormalities. Defects in the *FSHR* gene have been described but, since there is no alternative mechanism for follicular development in vivo, the distinction remains for the moment largely academic. The development of techniques to mature eggs in vitro to a fertilisable condition may make this a condition more amenable to treatment in the future.

POLYCYSTIC OVARY SYNDROME

PCOS can be considered an entirely separate condition from those described above. Originally described by Stein and Leventhal in 1935, it is characterised by obesity, oligo- or amenorrhoea, and hirsutism. This classic triad of symptoms is seen in many but not all women with PCOS and making a diagnosis in recent years has been contentious. It is recognised that there are a range of symptoms and signs from polycystic-appearing ovaries on ultrasound scan through to the full-blown Stein–Leventhal syndrome. In 2003, however, the Revised Rotterdam

Consensus provided clear diagnostic criteria based on the presence of two out of three of the following:

- polycystic-appearing ovaries on ultrasound scan
- oligo- or amenorrhoea
- either biochemical or clinical evidence of hyperandrogenism.

Other problems aside, women with PCOS who are oligo- or amenorrhoeic fail to ovulate regularly or to ovulate at all. They do, however, have functional ovaries that could potentially be made to ovulate. The polycystic appearance is the result of a large number (more than 12) of small antral follicles (2–9 mm) typically, but not exclusively, arranged around the periphery of the structure (a pearl necklace appearance) in at least one enlarged ovary. These antral follicles each produce a small amount of estrogen but they are effectively arrested at that stage of maturity. This continuous estrogen secretion means that women with PCOS anovulation are not estrogen deficient. Unopposed estrogen causes proliferative growth of the endometrium and, without the progesterone-effected transition and subsequent hormone withdrawal and menses, this may result in dysfunctional or breakthrough bleeding, hyperplasia with or without atypia and ultimately endometrial cancer. Thus women with PCOS presenting with dysfunctional or disordered vaginal bleeding should be investigated with assessment of endometrial thickness usually by transvaginal ultrasound scan, and by endometrial biopsy if warranted.

The aetiology of PCOS is not fully understood and is multifactorial. There is a genetic element, with frequent evidence of a family history of the disorder, and a racial element, with higher frequency and more severe effects in women from the Indian subcontinent, for example. There is also a known environmental effect of diet and weight. While there are slim women with PCOS, it appears that increasing body weight can exacerbate the severity of the syndrome and can on occasion be responsible for the development of the syndrome in women who, when lighter, would not have met the diagnostic criteria. PCOS is associated with developing insulin resistance and it is this relationship and associated metabolic syndrome that appears to contribute to ovarian functional arrest, perhaps through the mediation of insulin and insulin-like growth factors and their effects on follicular thecal cells. A consequent increase in ovarian androgen secretion results in a reduction in sex hormone-binding globulin (SHBG) synthesis in the liver such that free circulating androgens, including testosterone, are effectively increased. This, in turn, contributes to alterations in pituitary gonadotrophin secretion, with an increase in LH relative to FSH. Both then work to maintain the ovarian changes and set up a cycle of dysfunction of the whole hypothalamic–pituitary–ovarian axis, resulting in long-term anovulation if untreated. The key to management of anovulation is to break that vicious cycle either by stimulating changes in the hormone cycle or by removing the metabolic drivers.

Investigation and diagnosis

HISTORY

History and examination of women presenting with infertility is discussed elsewhere. In those presenting with anovulation, it is important to be aware that they are at risk of a number of associated conditions that should be specifically sought (Table 3.2).

Table 3.2 Anovulation – associated conditions

WHO classification	Symptoms	Associated problems
Group 1	Primary amenorrhoea: failure to enter puberty Secondary amenorrhoea: hot flushes, decreased libido, vaginal dryness, skin and hair changes	Underlying pituitary tumour, underlying eating disorder, osteoporosis, infertility, cardiovascular risk
Group 2	Secondary oligo- or amenorrhoea, dysfunctional uterine bleeding, obesity, hirsutism and acne, male pattern balding	Infertility, endometrial hyperplasia, endometrial adenocarcinoma, insulin resistance, type 2 diabetes, metabolic syndrome, increased cardiovascular risk
Group 3	As for Group 1	Osteoporosis, infertility, cardiovascular risk, underlying gonadal dysgenesis with its medical sequelae

BMI should be calculated in all anovulatory women since both high and low BMI may be associated and potentially causative features. At first presentation of primary amenorrhoea, however, it is important to establish the presence of secondary sexual characteristics and the absence of structural abnormalities of the gynaecological tract. In women with PCOS, the extent of hirsutes should be assessed (the Ferriman–Gallwey score is a useful tool for this) and stigmata of the metabolic syndrome sought, such as acanthosis nigricans. Examination may also reveal clues to other less common diagnoses such as Cushing syndrome, with the appearance of livid striae and typical facies, which might otherwise be mistaken for PCOS.

INVESTIGATIONS

Pelvic imaging, which is often undertaken at the time of examination by transvaginal ultrasound scan, can confirm normal pelvic organs and also provide an assessment of ovarian morphology, in particular polycystic appearance. In anovulatory PCOS, assessment of the endometrial thickness is also of benefit when considering the risk of hyperplasia. Significant thickening unaltered by progesterone-induced menses warrants further assessment, initially at least by endometrial biopsy.

A battery of endocrine, blood and other tests may be undertaken to reach a diagnosis (Table 3.3). Primary investigations may be completed together to expedite diagnosis but are not exhaustive and further (secondary) tests will be appropriate to specific conditions or related to specific treatment plans.

Table 3.3   Investigation of ovulatory disorders

Purpose	Primary investigation	Secondary investigation
Exclude pregnancy	Serum hCG	
Possible prolactinoma	Serum prolactin	MRI/CT if prolactin > 1000 mU/l
Assess for hypoestrogenism	Estradiol	If basal, assess for Group 1 or 3 If not basal, assess for Group 2, usually PCOS
Distinction between ovarian (Group 3) or hypothalamic–pituitary (Group 1) problem	FSH and LH	If increased, assess for primary ovarian insufficiency If low/normal, consider hypothalamic influences If basal, consider further pituitary assessment
Assess for PCOS (Group 2)	Testosterone or free androgen index (testosterone : SHBG ratio) TVUS for ovarian morphology	Urinalysis for glucose Lipid profile Random blood glucose Consider OGTT TVUS assessment of endometrial thickness
Assess for other Group 2 disorders such as late-onset adrenal hyperplasia	17-hydroxyprogesterone (17OHP)	
Assessment of primary ovarian insufficiency (Group 3)	FSH LH Estradiol AMH TVUS for AFC	Karyotype including *FMR1* analysis for fragile X syndrome Autoimmune antibodies (thyroid autoantibodies minimum)
Other, usually based on clinical findings	TSH for thyroid disorders	Cortisol (Cushing syndrome)

AFC = antral follicle count; AMH = antimüllerian hormone; CT = computed tomography; FSH = follicle-stimulating hormone; hCG = human chorionic gonadotrophin; LH = luteinising hormone; MRI = magnetic resonance imaging; OGTT = oral glucose tolerance test; SHBG = sex hormone-binding globulin; TSH = thyroid-stimulating hormone; TVUS = transvaginal ultrasound

OTHER FERTILITY CONSIDERATIONS

Semen analysis for the male partner must be considered an absolute minimum. It is important to consider tubal patency if ovulation induction is planned and, in women with risk factors for tubal disease, prior assessment should be considered mandatory either by laparoscopy or contrast imaging (hysterosalpingography [HSG] or hysterosalpingo-contrast-sonography [HyCoSy]). In women with no risk factors, it is acceptable to defer this invasive test, undertaking it if no pregnancy ensues after a limited number of ovulations have been achieved.

Liaison with medical and endocrinology specialists

Liaison with endocrine colleagues is recommended when more complex endocrine disorders are involved, such as when a pituitary tumour is suspected, although these may already been diagnosed and managed in that setting. Similarly, a woman with Turner syndrome may readily conceive with egg donation treatment but requires cardiac work-up before pregnancy to ensure that she is fit to do so. Fertility management cannot be viewed in isolation.

Treatment

General fertility advice is important, including advice (for both partners) on weight management, smoking, alcohol and drugs, as is confirming an up-to-date smear result and female folic acid supplementation.

WEIGHT MANAGEMENT

For women who are overweight (BMI $> 25 \text{kg/m}^2$) or especially if obese (BMI $> 30 \text{kg/m}^2$) and particularly those with a diagnosis of PCOS, the first line of management must always be for them to lose weight. In some women, normal menses will resume even before a target weight is reached. This is particularly likely in women who have previously been known to have regular menstrual cycles at a lower BMI. The advantages of this approach are two-fold: the risks associated with a future pregnancy are reduced significantly; and, even if the woman fails to ovulate as her weight decreases, she is more likely to respond to drug treatment. It is not recommended that women attempt to conceive or undergo fertility treatment during times of rapid weight loss because of the nutritional implications. This is an increasingly important scenario with the wider use of bariatric surgery being undertaken in women who are very obese.

DOPAMINE AGONISTS

In the case of microprolactinomas, treatment with a dopamine agonist is usually all that is required. Bromocriptine or cabergoline are the mainstays of treatment, acting to reduce prolactin production, relieving the gonadotrophin suppression and allowing resumption of the natural menstrual cycle. Under specialist supervision, it is appropriate to withdraw medication in pregnancy and reconsider its resumption after delivery, although both drugs are considered safe to be continued throughout pregnancy if necessary.

METFORMIN

Relief of the so-called metabolic syndrome may allow spontaneous cycles to resume. This may be achieved by weight loss alone but metformin was heralded as a medical holistic approach to the management of PCOS because of its role in the reduction of insulin resistance, which, it was hoped, would contribute to this process. However, current data have not yet confirmed the role of metformin as a single drug that can address all the pathological manifestations of PCOS. Metformin has been shown to increase the number of menses in women with PCOS but it has not shown significant benefit in weight loss or relief of other associated symptoms. Despite clinical variation in terms of the sample populations and drug regimens, aggregated data from trials comparing metformin with clomifene suggest that the two may be comparable in terms of live birth rates, while their combination may be more effective than either of them used on their own. It is still unclear as to whether there are pregnancy benefits in continuing metformin once conception is confirmed, and this is the focus on continuing trials.

CLOMIFENE AND TAMOXIFEN

Clomifene remains the mainstay of simple ovulation induction. It is cheap, easy to use and has few significant adverse effects. Clomifene is an anti-estrogen taken as a short 5-day course which, working at the level of the pituitary gland, enhances gonadotrophin production thus promoting the onset of follicular development and initiation of a cycle. It is dependent, therefore, on a functioning pituitary gland and may not be effective where there is a hypothalamic aetiology.

A programme of clomifene ovulation induction should be managed to provide the maximum chance of pregnancy at the lowest ovulatory dose possible over the shortest period. It is recommended that at least the first cycle be monitored by ultrasound scan to reduce the risk of inadvertent multi-folliculogenesis and multiple pregnancy, although high-order multiples are infrequent. Dose finding is usually undertaken in the range 50–150 mg daily although the maximum recommended dose is often 100 mg daily. Serious adverse effects are rare, with the most common complaints relating to follicular or corpus luteal cyst formation and premenstrual-type symptoms.

Clomifene has some negative effects on fertility (although the desired outcome of ovulation in anovulatory women outweighs these), namely thickening of cervical mucus potentially reducing sperm penetration, and alteration to the endometrium that may have an effect on implantation. There is a six-cycles' use licence limit on clomifene in the UK arising from data that suggested a link with ovarian cancer. Even though the original work relating to this has not been confirmed, the licence limit has been maintained. Although women requiring clomifene ovulation induction will often undertake more than six cycles of treatment in their reproductive lifetimes and should be informed of the concerns, most would consider the benefits largely outweigh the risks. Although ovarian hyperstimulation syndrome (OHSS) has been reported with clomifene use, it is rarely seen.

Anovulatory women with PCOS who commence a programme of clomifene treatment have a high chance (80%) of achieving ovulation and, if they ovulate, a 40% chance of pregnancy. Most women will conceive within six ovulatory cycles but there remains some gain in up to 12 cycles of treatment.

Tamoxifen has a similar mechanism of action but is less commonly used.

AROMATASE INHIBITORS

Aromatase inhibitors act by reducing the conversion of testosterone to estrogen. They are therefore capable of inducing ovulation by removing the negative feedback of estrogen on gonadotrophin secretion and, as with clomifene, promoting enough activity to initiate a cycle. The potential benefits of aromatase inhibitors over clomifene are that they do not suppress estrogen effects on the uterus and cervical mucus and therefore potentially may give higher success rates. Following the early closure of recruitment to a study of their use in the fertility setting because of a possible link with fetal abnormality, manufacturers withdrew from the fertility market and the drugs are only licensed for use in the UK in postmenopausal women. Nevertheless, research has continued and, as the original findings of a possible link with fetal abnormality have not been substantiated, there is increasing worldwide interest in these drugs as alternative ovulation induction agents.

GnRH ADMINISTRATION

Pulsatile GnRH administration is appropriate where pituitary function is normal. This includes women with PCOS. The advantage of this approach is the consequent physiological response of the pituitary and hence the ovaries such that multiple pregnancy risk and any concern of OHSS is reduced. GnRH has to be administered as a pulsatile infusion over several days or weeks and is therefore cumbersome and not widely accepted or offered.

GONADOTROPHIN STIMULATION

When the hypothalamus or pituitary gland is dysfunctional, FSH is administered in incrementally increasing doses to achieve ovarian stimulation – a so-called step-up regimen. The aim is for unifollicular ovulation at the lowest possible threshold; however, by virtue of the high antral follicle numbers available, particularly in women with PCOS, this is not always achievable, leading to an increased risk of multiple pregnancy or cycle cancellation. OHSS is a widely quoted but uncommon complication of this treatment because, while multi-follicular development remains a possibility, advances in the understanding of protocols and in transvaginal ultrasound monitoring as well as a newer attitude to the risks of multiple pregnancy mean that cycles are potentially better controlled and cancellation a more acceptable outcome. These complications are thus less likely to occur. This recognition also makes the use of GnRH agonists, previously rejected as it was considered that they increased the risk of OHSS, more acceptable adjuncts, their use avoiding premature or uncontrolled ovulation.

Gonadotrophin stimulation is also a suitable second-line management option for women with PCOS who fail to ovulate with maximum doses of clomifene.

FOLLICLE REDUCTION AND IN VITRO FERTILISATION

In women with a finite number of excess follicles at ovulation induction, it is possible to reduce the number of oocytes available for ovulation by means of follicle reduction. Transvaginal oocyte retrieval removes the excess such that sperm delivery, either by natural intercourse or by intrauterine insemination (IUI), may result in pregnancy with a reduced multiples risk.

Ultimately, if ovarian stimulation is difficult to control, in vitro fertilisation (IVF) provides a suitable. if more complex. alternative. The advantage of this approach is that a cycle need not be cancelled in the presence of multiple follicular development, which is a positive outcome in IVF treatment. Care needs to be taken when following IVF stimulation protocols in women with PCOS to avoid gross excess follicular development and a resultant high risk of OHSS. In women who have failed to conceive despite successful ovulation induction, it may be that there is another unexplained fertility factor and IVF may then be considered a treatment more likely to achieve successful pregnancy.

OVARIAN DRILLING

Ovarian drilling is an alternative to gonadotrophin administration in women with PCOS who are resistant to clomifene. It is a laparoscopic technique that is akin to the traditional ovarian wedge resection that is no longer practised. Four 4-second bursts of 40 W electrocautery to each ovary will, in a proportion of cases, cause ovulation to resume (50% with a conception rate of 40%), presumably by virtue of altering the intra-ovarian androgen balance, releasing antral follicles from their inhibitory influence. Spontaneous ovulation may not occur following ovarian drilling or may be short-lived. It is possible, however, that it may also enhance successful clomifene induction of ovulation. There remains some concern about the longer term effects of this destructive process although ovarian failure is rare and adhesion formation with low numbers of electrocautery points not significant.

EGG DONATION

For women with primary failure of ovarian function where oocytes are not available for ovulation induction, the only treatment option is oocyte donation. Although there are legal and ethical pitfalls that need to be considered, and egg donors are not easily recruited, this remains an effective and successful technique to allow pregnancy, childbirth and motherhood for suitable women. Where there are neither functional ovaries nor uterus, surrogacy may be considered.

Summary

Ovulatory disorders can arise from any level of the hypothalamic–pituitary–ovarian axis. Ovarian failure, which may be congenital or acquired, cannot be corrected but, if the rest of the reproductive tract is intact, egg donation is a possible route to pregnancy. Failure of the pathway at higher levels may be treated by correcting the underlying pathology (hyperprolactinaemia) or by stimulating an ovarian response medically. PCOS is a common and multifactorial condition that should be considered in its entirety, although it is often managed symptomatically. In PCOS, a surgical approach to ovulation induction is also a possibility.

OVULATORY DISORDERS: KEY LEARNING POINTS

- Understand the hypothalamic–pituitary–ovarian axis and the normal ovulatory menstrual cycle.
- Understand the main aetiologies of ovulatory disorders.
- Consider fertility problems as a couples issue and take other general health and fertility conditions into account.
- Understand the basis of assessment for ovulation dysfunction.
- Be able to apply appropriate investigations to make a diagnosis in ovulatory dysfunction.
- Understand the principles of fertility treatment in ovulatory dysfunction and their pitfalls.
- Consider when to engage with other specialists in the management of ovulatory dysfunction.
- Consider the syndrome of PCOS in conjunction with fertility issues.

Further reading

Arora P, Polson DW (2011) Diagnosis and management of premature ovarian failure. *The Obstetrician & Gynaecologist* 13: 67–72.

Balen AH (2008) *Metformin Therapy for the Management of Infertility in Women with Polycystic Ovary Syndrome.* Scientific Impact Paper No. 13. London: Royal College of Obstetricians and Gynaecologists.

Balen AH, Franks S, Homburg R, Kehoe S, editors (2010) *Current Management of Polycystic Ovary Syndrome.* London: RCOG Press.

Balen AH, Anderson RA (2007) Impact of obesity on female reproductive health: British Fertility Society Policy and Practice Guidelines. *Hum Fertil* 10: 195–206.

Bayram N, van Wely M, van der Ween F (2004) Pulsatile gonadotrophin releasing hormone for ovulation induction in subfertility associated with polycystic ovary syndrome. *Cochrane Database Syst Rev* (1):CD000412.

Farquhar C, Lilford RJ, Marjoribanks J, Vandekerckhove P (2007) Laparoscopic 'drilling' by diathermy or laser for ovulation induction in anovulatory polycystic ovary syndrome. *Cochrane Database Syst Rev* (3):CD001122. Update in *Cochrane Database Syst Rev* 2012;6:CD001122.

Homburg R (2005) *Ovulation Induction and Controlled Ovarian Stimulation: A Practical Guide.* London: Taylor & Francis.

Ledger W, Atkin SL, Cho LW (2007) *Long-term Consequences of Polycystic Ovary Syndrome.* Green-top Guideline No. 33. London: Royal College of Obstetricians and Gynaecologists.

Ledger W, Cheong Y (2011) *Reproductive Ageing*. Scientific Impact Paper No. 24. London: Royal College of Obstetricians and Gynaecologists.

Nugent D, Vandekerckhove P, Hughes E, Arnot M, Lilford R (2000) Gonadotrophin therapy for ovulation induction in subfertility associated with polycystic ovary syndrome. *Cochrane Database Syst Rev* (4):CD000410.

Tang T, Lord JM, Norman RJ, Yasmin E, Balen AH (2010) Insulin-sensitising drugs (metformin, rosiglitazone, pioglitazone, D-chiro-inositol) for women with polycystic ovary syndrome, oligo amenorrhoea and subfertility. *Cochrane Database Syst Rev* (1):CD003053. Update in: *Cochrane Database Syst Rev* 2012;5:CD003053.

4 Tubal infertility

Introduction

Fallopian tube damage accounts for 25–35% of infertility in women. In approximately three-quarters of cases the damage results from sexually transmitted infection (STIs) but tubal damage can also be as a result of pelvic surgery. The fallopian tubes play an essential role in conception, and tubal pathologies such as peritubal adhesions, proximal and/or distal tubal blockage, hydrosalpinx formation or endosalpingeal damage all have an adverse impact on fertility. The management of tubal disease depends on the initial pathological process and the severity of damage. In vitro fertilisation (IVF) remains the main treatment strategy for women with severely damaged fallopian tubes. Surgery can be useful in selected cases of tubal infertility and may have a complementary role for some women undergoing IVF. This chapter discusses these processes further but initially the basic anatomy of these remarkable but vulnerable structures is reviewed.

Anatomy

The fallopian tubes are derived from the müllerian ducts and are formed at the 6th week of embryological development. They comprise the isthmus, ampulla and infundibulum, with the latter's fimbrial end essential for picking up an ovum from the rupturing ovarian follicle. Each tube is about 10 cm long (range 7–14 cm). The lumen varies in diameter from 0.1 mm at the isthmus to 1 cm at the distal end of the ampulla. The columnar epithelium lining the tubes includes two different cell types: ciliated cells concentrated at the distal end of the tube and secretory cells at the ampullary region. The tubal cilia and peristaltic contractions of the tubal muscles transport the ovum to the uterus over 3–4 days while tubal secretions provide the essential environment for fertilisation.

Gross anatomical damage to the tubes is obvious in the case of a hydrosalpinx (Figure 4.1) although more subtle damage to the intricate tubal mucosa can be difficult to assess macroscopically.

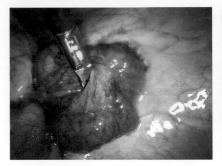

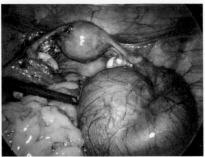

Figure 4.1a A normal fimbrial end of a fallopian tube during laparoscopy

Figure 4.1b A right hydrosalpinx

Aetiology

The main causes of tubal factor infertility include previous tubal infection, previous surgery, endometriosis and congenital abnormalities.

INFECTION

Fallopian tube functions can be affected through disruption of the delicate fimbriae or the inner mucosal micro-architecture. *Chlamydia trachomatis*, *Neisseria gonorrhoeae*, *Escherichia coli*, mycoplasma, *Bacteroides ureolyticus* and species of mobiluncus are known to cause deciliation and/or reduced ciliary activity. Pelvic inflammatory disease can result from unprotected sexual intercourse but also as a complication of miscarriage, termination of pregnancy, surgical procedures and investigations involving the uterine cavity, puerperal sepsis or the insertion of an intrauterine contraceptive device. In the above scenarios, clinicians should consider screening for infection or giving prophylactic antibiotics to at-risk groups.

Between 50% and 70% of tubal factor infertility is the result of *Chlamydia trachomatis* infection. Repeated and/or persistent chlamydial infections are particularly associated with pathology leading to pelvic adhesions, tubal scarring and occlusion. As many as 70% of chlamydial infections are asymptomatic and many women presenting with infertility will not be aware of a previous infection. Safer sex campaigns and the introduction of the National Chlamydia Screening Programme in 2003 were aimed at reducing the burden of tubal damage. The estimated rate of screening in 2008–09 of the target population group was 24%. A model developed by the Health Protection Agency indicated that testing 26–43% of the 16- to 24-year-old population could be expected to produce a substantial reduction in the prevalence of chlamydial infection. It is not yet known how the programme will impact on the long-term complication rates.

Another organism implicated in pelvic inflammatory disease is the Gram-negative diplococcus *Neisseria gonorrhoeae*. In recent years, the number of reported cases of gonorrhoea has continued to increase. As with *Chlamydia trachomatis*, many infected women will remain asymptomatic, but 50% present with vaginal discharge. Gonococci invade the non-ciliated cells of the tubal mucosa but predominantly destroy the ciliated cells primarily by causing sloughing.

Pelvic infection secondary to *Actinomyces israelli* is a rare complication of intrauterine contraceptive devices. As these devices tend to be used in older parous women, there is little in the literature regarding pelvic actinomycosis and infertility.

The majority of infections discussed above involve ascending microorganisms from the vagina and cervix to the endometrial cavity and then bilaterally into the fallopian tubes. Adjacent inflammatory processes such as appendicitis or a Crohn's disease abscess may affect the fallopian tubes by direct extension of the inflammatory process from the site of infection.

In developing countries, tuberculosis is a common cause of infertility. Genital tuberculosis affects about 12% of patients with pulmonary tuberculosis. In India, up to 19% of women with infertility have genital tuberculosis. Diagnosis involves a high index of suspicion when assessing women from high-prevalence areas.

SURGERY

Adhesions can form secondary to infection and/or inflammation, and they are often also a consequence of peritoneal injury after surgery. Adhesions can result in mechanical distortion of tubo-ovarian anatomy and direct blockage of the distal ends of the fallopian tubes. While adhesions external to the fallopian tubes can be lysed surgically, intra-tubal adhesions are not easily amenable to surgical treatment.

The peritoneum consists of a layer of mesothelial cells loosely connected to a basement membrane. During intraoperative tissue handling, the mesothelial cells are easily disrupted from their attachments to the basement membrane. Injury to the peritoneum leads to a cascade of events involving the cellular and fibrinolytic pathways to repair the damage over 7 days. The end result can be healthy peritoneal tissue with no adhesions. However, in the presence of a foreign body, tissue ischaemia or when two injured peritoneal surfaces are opposed, the fibrinolytic process is inhibited. The matrix of inflammatory exudate and primitive mesothelial cells gradually reorganises and becomes replaced by tissue-containing fibroblasts and inflammatory cells. Fibrin bands form and reorganise into adhesions.

Reported incidences of postoperative adhesions after gynaecological surgery range from 50% to 90% and should be considered as a potential cause of tubal damage in women who have undergone abdominal and pelvic surgery. Good surgical technique with minimal handling of tissue and meticulous attention to haemostasis can reduce the risk of adhesion formation. Over the years various pharmacological and therapeutic interventions have been trialled to see whether adhesion formation can be reduced but none of the studies have specifically examined adhesion prevention with respect to peritubal adhesions and fertility.

ENDOMETRIOSIS

Pelvic endometriosis can result in distortion and blockage of the fallopian tubes. Studies have also shown that the level of activated macrophages in the peritoneal cavity is raised in endometriosis, which has a detrimental effect on ciliary beat frequency and peristaltic action of the fallopian tubes and uterus. This topic is reviewed in Chapter 5.

CONGENITAL ABNORMALITIES

Congenital abnormalities are rare but may include:

- aplasia, in which the tube fails to form
- hypoplasia, in which the tube is long, tortuous and narrow
- accessory ostia or congenital diverticula.

Pathology

Infection, endometriosis and surgery affect tubal function via different mechanisms but all lead to inflammation. The basic characteristics of inflammation are always the same.

ACUTE INFLAMMATION

Acute inflammation involves dynamic changes in blood vessels, blood flow and leucocytosis. If the inflammatory response destroys or neutralises the causative agent without significant local tissue damage, resolution with restoration of normal anatomy occurs. With tissue destruction, there will be regeneration or organisation. The ultimate result depends on a balance between these two processes.

CHRONIC INFLAMMATION

Chronic inflammation involves mononuclear blood cells. Proliferating fibroblasts and capillaries represent repair by organisation. Granulomatous chronic inflammation is a variant where macrophages predominate in multiple, small, discrete, concentric aggregates (granulomata). Around this mass of macrophages is a cuff of lymphocytes, often with granulation tissue and, later on in all lesions, fibrosis.

Infection and inflammation of the fallopian tubes can therefore result in intra-tubal pathology as well as extra-tubal adhesions, both of which contribute to infertility. Intraluminal adhesions can lead to partial obstruction and the risk of ectopic pregnancy. Complete and chronic obstruction leads to fluid collection in the distal portion of the fallopian tube; that is, a hydrosalpinx. Peritubal and periovarian adhesions can be divided surgically but intra-tubal mucosal damage is irreversible. The management of adhesions and hydrosalpinx is discussed later in this chapter.

Infection screening of high-risk groups

Women with tubal damage may present with subfertility to their GP. Access to cost-effective screening techniques to detect those at high risk of tubal damage who may require secondary care input is desirable. Taking an endocervical swab or first-catch urine sample for chlamydia may be useful although this strategy only helps identify current infection. Infection with *Chlamydia trachomatis* results in the formation of antibodies detectable in the serum. Chlamydia serology may be useful in identifying women with a previous history of infection and titres may have predictive value in detecting the presence and severity of tubal damage.

Investigations and diagnosis

DIAGNOSTIC TECHNIQUES AVAILABLE FOR ASSESSING TUBAL DISEASE

In the context of subfertility, before assessing tubal patency both semen analysis and assessment of ovulation should be carried out. It is also essential that high-risk women be screened for chlamydia. The recommendation in the National Institute for Health and Care Excellence (NICE) *Fertility* guideline is for women without known comorbidities and at low risk of tubal compromise, to be offered hysterosalpingography (HSG) or, where the expertise is available, hysterosalpingo-contrast-sonography (HyCoSy). In women with a history of pelvic inflammatory disease, previous ectopic pregnancy or symptoms suggestive of endometriosis, a laparoscopy and dye should be offered.

HYSTEROSALPINGOGRAPHY

HSG is a simple, safe and inexpensive X-ray-based contrast study of the uterine cavity and fallopian tubes (Figure 4.2). HSG has a high specificity (a low false-positive rate) but lower sensitivity (a relatively high false-negative rate) for detecting tubal blockage. Imaging should be performed during the follicular phase of the menstrual cycle when the endometrium is thin and when pregnancy has been excluded. Features looked for on an HSG include:

- the presence of proximal tubal disease (salpingitis isthmica nodosa, polyps)
- ampullary mucosal folds (a healthy sign)
- filling defects inside the ampulla suggestive of fibrosis
- tubal dilatation
- tubal patency or obstruction
- loculation of medium.

Caution should be taken of diagnosing false tubal occlusion secondary to tubal spasm or endometrial debris.

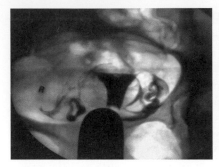

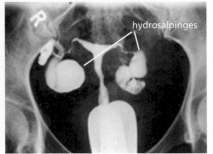

Figure 4.2a HSG showing normal patency of the fallopian tubes

Figure 4.2b Abnormal HSG with bilateral hydrosalpinges

HYSTEROSALPINGO-CONTRAST-SONOGRAPHY

HyCoSy is a simple procedure that uses ultrasound. A sonoreflective echo-contrast fluid is introduced into the uterine cavity allowing assessment of the outline of the uterine cavity and the patency of the fallopian tubes. Echovist® (Schering Health Care, Burgess Hill, West Sussex) consists of a suspension of micron-sized air bubbles, formed upon reconstitution of specially formulated galactose granules with an aqueous galactose solution. These microbubbles are extremely echogenic and create a very bright echo, even in the very narrow lumen of the fallopian tube, and this can be visualised on ultrasound.

The advantages of this technique are that it is inexpensive, safe, almost 100% sensitive (no false negatives), allows simultaneous assessment of the ovaries with ultrasound and provides an instant result seen by the patient. The specificity is only in the region of 75% so women with a positive test should be offered a laparoscopy. In 2004, a survey found that only 14% of UK clinics used HyCoSy. This is because the learning curve is steep and the procedure is very operator dependent.

LAPAROSCOPY AND DYE STUDIES

Surgery via laparoscopy and dye hydrotubation allows concurrent assessment of the ovaries and the peritoneum. One significant advantage of surgery is that pelvic pathology can be concomitantly treated. Methylene blue dye, which is used for hydrotubation, very rarely causes allergic or other adverse reactions. The overall risk of complications from a diagnostic laparoscopy is approximately one in 500, so surgery should only be performed when indicated.

The therapeutic effect of flushing the fallopian tubes and the potential clearing of obstruction has been debated for half a century. In 2007, Johnson et al. published a randomised controlled trial (RCT) comparing lipiodol (a poppy seed oil) flushing with no intervention. They found a significant benefit in pregnancy rate following lipiodol flushing. A larger multicentre RCT is under way to confirm the results.

SPECIALIST TECHNIQUES

Salpingoscopy involves introducing an endoscope via the fimbrial end of the fallopian tube to visualise the internal tubal mucosa at the time of laparoscopy. Tubal pathology is then classified based on the extent of macroscopic mucosal damage. Some studies have suggested that salpingoscopy may be a useful tool in predicting future pregnancy but it is not a routinely performed technique.

Falloposcopy is a technique where an endoscope is introduced to the tube trans-cervically. A guidewire is inserted through the cervix over which a catheter is passed. The endoscope is then passed through the catheter, allowing the surgeon to visualise the full length of the internal mucosa. If obstruction is identified, balloon dilation can be used to correct the problem. There are currently no RCTs of falloposcopy and technical problems limit the use of this procedure in routine clinical practice.

Classification of tubal disease

Classification of tubal disease is essential for use in clinical trials but also as a potential prognostic indicator to assist patients and clinicians in decisions regarding further management. There is no single, universally agreed classification system for scoring tubal damage. The 'Hull and Rutherford' (H&R) classification, which was published in 2002, was based on assessment of the fallopian tubes made mainly at laparoscopy complemented by findings from HSG. Tubal surgical repair using microsurgical techniques during open surgery achieved live birth rates of 69%, 48% and 9% for grades I, II and III, respectively, over a 10-year study period. This classification system can distinguish women into three distinct groups giving a favourable, fair and poor prognosis for pregnancy following tubal surgery. However, there can be a wide variation of damage within each group and the assessment is subjective.

HULL AND RUTHERFORD CLASSIFICATION OF TUBAL DISEASE	
Grade I – minor	Tubal fibrosis absent even if tube occluded (proximally) Tubal distension absent even if tube occluded (distally) Mucosal appearances favourable Adhesions (peritubal – ovarian) are flimsy
Grade II – intermediate or moderate	Unilateral severe tubal disease (see below) with or without contra-lateral minor damage 'Limited' dense adhesions of tubes and/or ovaries
Grade III – severe	Bilateral tubal damage Tubal fibrosis extensive Tubal distension > 1.5 cm Abnormal mucosal appearance Bipolar occlusion 'Extensive' dense adhesions

Management options also depend on the site of occlusion, so classification can also be anatomical, dividing tubal occlusion into proximal, midtubal and distal:

- Proximal tubal occlusion can be due to mucus plugs, cornual synechiae, polyps or tubal endometriosis. However, the most common histopathological finding of true cornual occlusion is salpingitis isthmica nodosa. The characteristics of salpingitis isthmica nodosa are the presence of diverticula of the tubal epithelium that are surrounded by hypertrophied smooth muscle. The cause of salpingitis isthmica nodosa is not always clear but it may in some cases be a congenital defect, or it could be a result of acute or chronic inflammation due to infection. Proximal obstruction occurs in 10–25% of women with tubal disease.

- Midtubal occlusion is usually iatrogenic from tubal sterilisation.

- Distal tubal occlusion is related to salpingitis secondary to any pelvic inflammatory condition including infection, endometriosis, appendicitis and abdomino-pelvic surgery. Distal inflammation leading to occlusion results in accumulation of a watery discharge and formation of a hydrosalpinx.

Management options: prognostic factors

Once tubal disease has been identified, management options include expectant management, tubal cannulation, surgery and IVF. Several prognostic factors need to be considered when counselling women regarding their individual further management options.

AGE

The success rates associated with tubal surgery as well as assisted conception are influenced by the age of the woman and the duration of follow-up. One study quoted conception rates after surgery at the end of 50 months of 27% for women aged 21–25 years, 38% for those aged 26–30 years, 32% for those aged 31–35 years and 36% for those aged 36 years and above. The conception rate for women over 40 was not separately assessed in this study. This needs to be compared with the couples' predicted chances of conception following IVF. The national statistics from the Human Fertilisation and Embryology Authority (HFEA) for the UK in 2008 (published in 2011) showed that the live birth rates per cycle of IVF for the various age groups were as follows: 33.1% (< 35 years), 27.2% (35–37 years), 19.3% (38–39 years), 12.5% (40–42 years), 10.6% (40–42 years) and 3.2% (>42 years). While it is clear that IVF can help women with tubal disease achieve a pregnancy in a shorter time, other factors such as availability and affordability of IVF play a significant part in the final clinical decision for treatment.

CAUSE, TYPE AND SEVERITY OF TUBAL DISEASE

When assessing the outcome of surgery, the location and severity of damage appears to be the most important prognostic factor rather than the cause of tubal damage. The chance of pregnancy after surgery is significantly better in women with mild to moderate disease compared with those with severe disease. The surgical removal of hydrosalpinges is required to enhance the success rate of IVF. This is discussed later in the chapter.

It is possible that women with moderate or severe endometriosis who also have tubal disease are more likely to benefit from surgery than those who do not have tubal damage from the endometriosis.

Treatment

TUBAL SURGERY

The main surgical options for tubal damage include adhesiolysis, fimbrioplasty, salpingostomy, tubo-tubal re-anastomosis and salpingectomy. The preferred route for many surgeons is laparoscopic. Detailed descriptions of tubal surgery techniques are beyond the scope of this book though brief descriptions of fimbrioplasty and salpingostomy follow below. Both are performed with meticulous attention to haemostasis.

When the distal tube is damaged, a ring of scar tissue can form that compresses and enfolds the fimbriae. A fimbrioplasty involves excising the fibrous tissue and dividing the mucosal bridge and then everting the mucosal edges.

Salpingostomy is performed for distal obstruction and involves creating a new tubal opening with exaggerated eversion of the opening to expose healthy mucosa.

Tubo-tubal re-anastomosis is usually performed for reversal of sterilisation, and this is discussed later in this chapter.

SURGERY VERSUS IVF

Couples with infertility resulting from tubal disease have two therapeutic options: reconstructive tubal surgery or IVF. Tubal microsurgery is a recognised treatment for tubal infertility but intrauterine pregnancy rates after surgery are on average only 25% per year compared with pregnancy rates of over 30% after one cycle of IVF. A successful tubal repair gives women the possibility of conceiving more than once without further treatment, as well as the psychological advantage of being able to conceive spontaneously. The downside is the increased risk of ectopic pregnancy after tubal surgery and an ultrasound scan should be performed early on to confirm the pregnancy site.

Table 4.1 lists issues that need to be discussed with couples trying to decide between IVF and tubal surgery. While the available evidence is a key factor that should inform the counselling process, there are also important logistical and psychological factors that need to be considered.

Table 4.1 Tubal surgery versus IVF – issues to be discussed with couples

Issue	IVF	Tubal surgery
Availability on the NHS	If certain criteria are met (see local primary care trust guidelines; varies from area to area)	Where the expertise is available, and in carefully selected women
Privately funded cost	£5000–6000 for one cycle[a]	£3000–4000[a] but available on the NHS in general
Time off work	1–2 days	5 days to 6 weeks
Multiple hospital visits	Yes	No
Requires administration of hormones	Yes	No
Success rates (live birth rates)	*By age.[b]* Under 35 years: 32.9% 35–40 years: 19–27% Over 40 years: 2–13%	*By Hull and Rutherford classification:* Minor: 69% Moderate: 48% Severe: 9%
Time after procedure until knowing whether successful	2 weeks	1–2 years or more
Risk of tubal pregnancy	1–2% of pregnancies	10–25% of pregnancies

IVF = in vitro fertilisation

[a] estimated cost based on local hospital figures in 2011

[b] these are averages; results are clinic dependent – see http://guide.hfea.gov.uk/guide/ for more detail

The authors of a Cochrane review in 2008 concluded that with the current research they were unable to determine the effectiveness or otherwise of tubal surgery compared with either IVF or expectant management. In practice, with IVF now widely available and fewer surgeons with substantive experience in microsurgery, the management of tubal factor infertility is, for the most part, appropriately confined to the use of IVF.

REVERSAL OF STERILISATION

When women are counselled regarding sterilisation they should be informed that it is considered a permanent form of contraception. Subsequent regret at loss of fertility occurs in 5–20% of women, though only a minority of them go on to request reversal. Reversal of sterilisation is often not available on the NHS. The success of tubal re-anastomosis depends on the initial sterilisation technique. When Filshie clips or Falope (Yoon's) rings were used, a return to fecundity is possible in approximately 80% of cases. However, if cautery methods were employed, the success rate is less than 50%. Success depends on the presence of at least a 5 cm portion of untraumatised tube. Reversal after hysteroscopic techniques of sterilisation is not achievable. When considering tubal re-anastomosis, the woman should be counselled regarding her likely personal success rate of IVF.

EXCISION OR OCCLUSION OF HYDROSALPINGES BEFORE IVF

Evidence suggests that IVF success rates are 50% lower in women with hydrosalpinges and blocked fallopian tubes. Studies suggest that the hydrosalpinx fluid may act on two different target systems: directly on the transferred embryo or on the endometrium and its receptivity for implantation, or both. Hydrosalpinx fluid lacks nutrients essential to the development of an embryo to a blastocyst. Hydrosalpinx fluid has also been found to have embryotoxic properties, with elevated concentrations of endotoxins, cytokines, microorganisms and oxidative and antioxidant systems. The presence of cytokines also affects the secretion and expression of cytokines and integrins essential for early embryo–endometrial interactions and implantation. Hydrosalpinx fluid has also been implicated in affecting endometrial peristalsis wave patterns and this could explain the reduced implantation rate.

Surgical treatment should be considered for all women with hydrosalpinges before IVF treatment. The management options for hydrosalpinges include drainage by ultrasound-guided aspiration, salpingostomy, salpingectomy and proximal tubal occlusion. A Cochrane review by Johnson et al. (2010) concluded that both laparoscopic salpingectomy and tubal occlusion before IVF increase the odds of pregnancy. Further research is required to assess the value of drainage by aspiration.

TUBAL INFERTILITY: KEY POINTS

- Tubal damage accounts for 25–35% of infertility in women.
- 50–70% of tubal factor infertility is a result of chlamydia.
- All surgeons operating on women of childbearing age need to ensure that they pay particular attention to preventing adhesions.
- IVF and tubal surgery are complementary but IVF is increasingly being used as the treatment of choice for tubal factor infertility.

Further reading

Akande VA, Cahill DJ, Wardle PG, Rutherford AJ, Jenkins JM (2004) The predictive value of the "Hull & Rutherford" classification for tubal damage. *BJOG* 111:1236–41.

Akande VA, Hunt LP, Cahill DJ, Caul EO, Ford WC, Jenkins JM (2003) Tubal damage in infertile women: prediction using chlamydia serology. *Hum Reprod* 18:1841–7.

Johnson N, van Voorst S, Sowter MC, Strandell A, Mol BW (2010) Surgical treatment for tubal disease in women due to undergo in vitro fertilisation. *Cochrane Database Syst Rev* (1):CD002125.

Johnson NP, Kwok R, Stewart AW, Saththianathan M, Hadden WE, Chamley LW (2007) Lipiodol fertility enhancement: two-year follow-up of a randomized trial suggests a transient benefit in endometriosis, but a sustained benefit in unexplained infertility. *Hum Reprod* 22:2857–62.

Metwally M, Watson A, Lilford R, Vandekerckhove P (2006) Fluid and pharmacological agents for adhesion prevention after gynaecological surgery. *Cochrane Database Syst Rev* (2):CD001298.

National Collaborating Centre for Women's and Children's Health, National Institute for Health and Clinical Excellence (2013) *Fertility: Assessment and Treatment for People with Fertility Problems.* 2nd ed. London: Royal College of Obstetricians and Gynaecologists [http://guidance.nice.org.uk/CG156/Guidance].

Singhal V, Li TC, Cooke ID (1991) An analysis of factors influencing the outcome of 232 consecutive tubal microsurgery cases. *Br J Obstet Gynaecol* 98:628–36.

Pandian Z, Akande VA, Harrild K, Bhattacharya S (2008) Surgery for tubal infertility. *Cochrane Database Syst Rev* (3):CD006415.

Vyjayanthi S, Kingsland CR, Dunham R, Balen AH (2004) National survey of current practice in assessing tubal patency in the UK. *Hum Fertil* 7:267–70.

5 Endometriosis-related infertility

Introduction

Endometriosis causes pain and infertility for millions of women worldwide. Although first reported by Rokitansky 150 years ago, debate continues over its aetiology, pathogenesis and most effective treatment.

Aetiology

Endometriosis may be defined as the presence and proliferation of endometrial-like tissue outside the uterus, primarily on the pelvic peritoneum, ovaries and rectovaginal septum. The prevalence (proportion of women with the disease at any one time) of endometriosis is 6–10% in women of reproductive age, and 30–50% of women with pelvic pain and/or infertility.

The most widely accepted theory of pathogenesis is Sampson's 'transplantation theory'. Sampson proposed that retrograde flow of endometrial cells from the uterine cavity, through the fallopian tubes, into the pelvic cavity during menstruation deposits viable tissue that implants on the peritoneal surface. This theory is supported by data showing an increased occurrence of endometriosis in women with müllerian duct anomalies causing genital outflow tract obstruction leading to increased retrograde menstruation. Women who menstruate more frequently, more heavily or for a longer duration, and therefore have increased exposure to retrograde menstruation, also have a higher risk of developing the disease. Additional risk factors include prolonged exposure to estrogen (such as in early menarche and late menopause), obesity, low birthweight and exposure to endocrine-disrupting chemicals. Twin and family studies suggest a genetic component. Prolonged breastfeeding and higher numbers of pregnancies are protective.

Although 90% of women have retrograde flow during menses, only 6–10% develop endometriosis. These data suggest that women with endometriosis either have a different type of endometrium, which is more likely to implant and proliferate following retrograde menstruation, and/or that affected women have a failure in their immune mechanisms that should prevent peritoneal implantation of the ectopic tissue. Recent studies suggest that both of these factors are likely to be true. It appears that the endometrium (that is, the eutopic endometrium lining the endometrial cavity) is altered in women with endometriosis in a number of ways:

- abnormal, inflammation-related, in situ production of estradiol
- resistance to the effects of progesterone
- increased numbers of macrophages, dendritic cells and consequently cytokines
- the presence of nerve fibres in the functional layer of the endometrium.

Ovarian suppression with gonadotrophin-releasing hormone (GnRH) analogues or oral contraceptives corrects these alterations. Retrograde menstrual tissue collected from the pelvis at surgery implants and proliferates in vitro more rapidly when it originates from women with endometriosis compared with unaffected patients.

However, other theories are also needed to explain the occasional presence of endometriosis in sites distant from the female pelvis: for example, in the pleural cavity, central nervous system, and, in a few isolated cases, the male prostate. It has been proposed that lymphatic or haematogenous spread, metaplasia of peritoneal mesothelium, or the development of endometriosis from embryonic rests could explain these findings. It is generally accepted that retrograde menstruation probably causes most of the cases of endometriosis.

Pathophysiology

The two most common disorders associated with endometriosis are infertility and pain. However, there is limited correlation between the extent of disease and the degree of pain and/or fertility problems. The most commonly used way of objectively staging the severity of endometriosis is that described by the American Society for Reproductive Medicine. Following visual assessment of the pelvis at surgery, a weighted score is calculated based on the number, size, position and depth of endometrial implants, and the presence and type of adhesions. Arbitrary cut-off values divide the disease into minimal, mild, moderate and severe grades.

The classic endometriotic implant is the blue-black 'powder-burn' lesion, although the disease can also appear in more subtle forms including red or white lesions (Figure 5.1). The inflammatory nature of the deposits leads to neovascular-

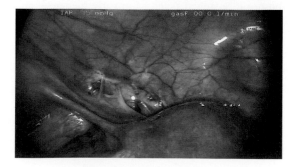

Figure 5.1 Endometriotic deposit and adhesions in uterovesical fold

isation and adhesion formation. Implants of endometriosis on the surface of the ovary can, ultimately, lead to invagination and the formation of an endometriotic cyst known as an endometrioma. These cysts have a wall formed by endometriotic tissue and contain dark, thick cystic fluid; hence their other name, 'chocolate cysts'.

Endometriosis is considered to be a cause of infertility. This theory is based on observations of higher prevalence of endometriosis in infertile women. Although this does not prove causation, it is accepted that endometriosis severe enough to distort pelvic anatomy is associated with reduced fecundity.

The effect of minimal or mild endometriosis on fertility is less clear. Support for a link comes from cohort studies where women undergoing artificial insemination with peritoneal endometriosis had lower pregnancy rates than those with no endometriosis. A Cochrane review of randomised controlled trials (RCTs) evaluating the benefit of surgery in women with minimal or mild endometriosis has confirmed that treatment results in improved fertility. It has been suggested that such disease may have an adverse effect through the raised levels of growth and inflammatory factors found in the peritoneal fluid of women with endometriosis. Since oocyte fertilisation normally takes place within the ampulla of the fallopian tube, which is exposed to the abnormal peritoneal fluid, it is feasible that natural conception could be affected. The inflammatory changes in the peritoneal fluid include proliferation of macrophages and phagocytic dysfunction, and the release of proinflammatory and angiogenic factors. A number of studies have suggested that these peritoneal fluid abnormalities can adversely affect sperm motility, capacitation and sperm–oocyte binding.

In addition, the endometrium within the uterine cavity is different in women with endometriosis compared with those without, as described above. It is possible, though not proven, that the changes in endometrial function, particularly progesterone resistance, could adversely affect embryo implantation. This is supported by clinical data suggesting a higher embryo implantation rate in patients with endometriosis when in vitro fertilisation (IVF) follows prolonged ovarian suppression, which is recognised to normalise the uterine endometrial changes.

Both pelvic pain and dyspareunia due to endometriosis can affect a couple's ability to have regular sexual intercourse and so further reduce their fertility. Under these circumstances, surgery to remove endometriosis and improve both pain and fertility may have an important role.

The natural history of endometriosis is not well understood, although the disease does seem to progress in untreated women. However, regression of disease in 30–40% of women on second-look laparoscopy is well recognised in the placebo arm of RCTs. However, it is unclear to what extent early treatment can slow or halt disease progression.

Investigation and diagnosis

Endometriosis may be suggested by symptoms of pain and dyspareunia as well as a number of signs on physical examination of the pelvis. There may be tenderness and nodularity along the uterosacral ligaments and in the rectovaginal septum. The uterus may be fixed and retroverted and the ovaries may be enlarged and tender owing to the presence of endometriomas.

For definitive diagnosis and staging of endometriosis, a surgical procedure, generally a laparoscopy, is necessary to visualise disease implants. Occasionally, biopsy and histology of suspicious lesions is required. Surgical diagnosis also offers the option of treatment of lesions and/or adhesions at the same time; 'see and treat'.

Transvaginal ultrasound is able to diagnose ovarian endometriomas. Such cysts have a classic 'ground glass' appearance (Figure 5.2).

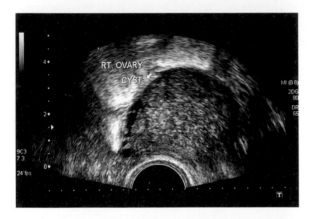

Figure 5.2 Transvaginal ultrasound scan of the pelvis showing an ovarian endometrioma

However, ultrasound is unable to visualise the more common superficial peritoneal disease. Movement of the ultrasound probe during transvaginal scanning can identify adnexal tenderness or fixed high ovaries that may suggest disease in that area. Areas of fluid collection around the ovaries can suggest peritoneal fluid trapped within adnexal adhesions. Hydrosalpinges suggest tubal blockage. All of these findings may be consistent with, but not diagnostic of, endometriosis.

More recently, magnetic resonance imaging (MRI) has been used as a non-invasive tool in the diagnosis of deep endometriosis. Although it has limitations in the visualisation of small endometriotic implants and adhesions, it can characterise the lesions, study extraperitoneal locations, examine the relationship of disease to other structures such as the ureters and bowel, and identify the contents of pelvic masses. MRI is also a sensitive test for diagnosing adenomyosis (also called endometriosis interna), in which endometrial tissue implants and proliferates within the myometrium. Adenomyosis is an under-diagnosed cause of pelvic pain, although it is not a cause of infertility.

Work continues on identifying useful biochemical diagnostic markers for endometriosis. Serum CA125 is often raised in endometriosis but has limited diagnostic utility owing to poor sensitivity and specificity.

Treatment

The aim of treatment of endometriosis is to remove or reduce disease deposits. This may be attempted through medical or surgical means. It has long been recognised that endometriotic glands are hormonally sensitive. Following observations of the improvement of endometriosis symptoms during pregnancy and after the menopause, medical regimens have been developed to mimic these physiological states. A pseudopregnancy state can be induced with the use of the oral contraceptive pill or continuous progestogens. A pseudomenopausal state is created by inducing anovulatory hypoestrogenism with drugs such as GnRH agonists or progestogens. The aim of these treatments is to induce atrophy within the hormonally dependent ectopic endometrium deposits so that they shrink in size and number. Two major problems with medical therapies are that, because of anovulation, conception is not possible during treatment and that treatment is prolonged, generally for 6 months. If pain is the only complaint, this is not important, but for subfertile women 6 months of iatrogenic infertility is generally unattractive. Management is correspondingly tailored to the relative importance to the woman of treating her pain or her fertility. If surgery is used, endometriotic deposits are fulgurated using diathermy, and excised or vaporised with scissors or laser.

EXPECTANT MANAGEMENT

Unless endometriosis is so severe that major distortion of the pelvic anatomy results, women with endometriosis are not completely infertile but may have a monthly conception rate below that of unaffected women. Consequently, one approach is for the couple to continue trying to conceive without undergoing active treatment; so-called 'expectant management'. As with all couples seen within the fertility clinic setting, advice should be given on optimising personal factors affecting fertility, particularly smoking and weight. The need for regular intercourse – ideally throughout the menstrual cycle, or at least around the time of ovulation – is emphasised. A full fertility work-up including semen analysis, confirmation of ovulation and tubal patency is undertaken. It is useful for couples to be offered a follow-up appointment so that they do not feel 'lost' in the system, and also to agree on a sensible timescale for expectant management before review and consideration of active treatment. The success of expectant management will clearly depend on a number of factors, particularly the woman's age, the severity of her endometriosis and the duration of infertility, as well as the presence of any associated male factor. Data from the ENDOCAN and Italian surgical trials, referred to below, show that women with untreated minimal or mild endometriosis had around a 23% chance of conceiving subsequently. Some of these women (around 10%) did, however, move on to active treatment during follow-up.

Expectant management will be most appropriate for women with minimal or mild endometriosis and is unlikely to benefit those with more severe disease.

MEDICAL TREATMENT

Current hormonal treatments for endometriosis, such as oral contraceptives, continuous progestogens and GnRH analogues, cause anovulation and so reduce the monthly conception rate during treatment to zero. Therefore, if therapy is to be of value in treating infertility, the post-treatment conception rate needs to be significantly increased. Unfortunately, a number of RCTs as well as a systematic review confirm that this is not the case. Consequently, these drugs should not be used for the treatment of infertility and should not delay the option of effective therapies.

SURGICAL TREATMENT

The aim of conservative surgery, appropriate for women with infertility, is to destroy endometriotic implants, remove endometriomas and divide adhesions so as to restore the pelvis to as near normal as possible. Ideally, such surgery is performed laparoscopically; however, laparotomy may have to be performed for removal of large endometriomas with extensive pelvic adhesions, when bowel involvement is severe, in the absence of suitable equipment, or where surgeons do not possess adequate laparoscopic training.

Few studies on surgery for endometriosis-related infertility are RCTs. Most publications are observational and of retrospective design, with all their inherent biases. Without knowing the effect on fecundity of no treatment in a control group, few concrete conclusions can be drawn. Unless severe disease has totally distorted the pelvis, most women with endometriosis are not totally infertile but continue to have a monthly conception rate. Consequently, expectant management could give fertility rates similar to or even better than those with surgery, particularly if the latter is destructive in nature.

In the ENDOCAN prospective, multicentre RCT that examined the efficacy of surgical treatment of minimal and mild endometriosis on infertility, 341 women were randomised and followed up for 36 weeks. The cumulative probabilities of pregnancy in the surgically treated and the non-treated groups were 30.7% and 17.7%, respectively (rate ratio 1.7; 95% CI 1.2–2.6). The implants and adhesions were treated with diathermy or laser, or a combination of the two. However, shortcomings of the study are that the patients were not blinded to the intervention received, approximately 10% of the women in each group received additional fertility medication or adhesiolysis, and the pregnancy rates in the control group were lower than expected (so potentially exaggerating the benefits of surgery). While a smaller Italian study with a similar design did not demonstrate any benefit of surgical treatment, a Cochrane systematic review combining the two studies did confirm that surgery improves outcome.

There is a lack of RCTs examining the role of surgery in fertility patients with moderate or severe endometriosis. It is generally considered that attempting to correct anatomical defects surgically should result in better outcomes than medical treatment or expectant management. However, this hypothesis has never been adequately tested.

It is believed that the medical treatment of endometriomas is ineffective. The value of surgical treatment of endometriomas compared with medical or expectant management for fertility has not been tested in a randomised setting. Conception rates of about 50% at 3 years after treatment, whether by laparoscopy or laparotomy, are reported. Without an untreated control group, it is not known what the rate would have been with expectant management. The two approaches to surgical removal of endometriomas are to open and drain the cyst and then either to strip the capsule away from the ovary or to attempt to ablate the capsule. RCTs have confirmed that stripping the capsule, compared with ablating, results in a lower rate of recurrence and a higher chance of natural conception. While the use of ovarian suppression with the contraceptive pill following ovarian cystectomy further reduces the recurrence rate, this approach is unlikely to be beneficial in the infertility setting.

Disadvantages of surgery involve the risks of the anaesthetic and the surgical procedure itself. A diagnostic laparoscopy is associated with a risk of two to three in 1000 of damaging internal structures. Women with moderate or severe endometriosis who undergo surgery to remove disease and/or adhesions are at increased risk of damage to their bladder, bowel, blood vessels and ureters. This risk needs to be weighed up against the likelihood of benefit in terms of improved fertility and reduced pelvic pain

It is clear that, for infertile couples with endometriosis, treatment options should include surgery. Medical treatments do not appear to increase fecundity. At some point, couples should be offered IVF treatment, as this gives the greatest chance of conception.

Assisted conception

Although assisted conception treatments such as ovulation induction with intrauterine insemination (IUI), or IVF, do not treat endometriosis per se, they can successfully treat the associated infertility. An RCT compared superovulation using gonadotrophins followed by IUI against no treatment for women with minimal or mild endometriosis. The IUI group had 14 live births out of 127 cycles (11%) compared with four out of 184 control cycles (2%). This gives an odds ratio for live birth of 5.6 (95% CI 1.8–17.4). However, stimulated IUI offers less control over the chance of multiple pregnancy compared with IVF since one cannot be sure how many of the developing follicles will ovulate. Increasingly, only a single embryo is replaced during IVF. In addition, the relatively low success rate of IUI, compared with IVF, means that its use is declining.

Age-related live birth rates after one cycle of IVF should be kept in mind when discussing treatment options. In particular, the reduction in IVF success as women pass through their mid to late 30s must be considered. If attempting surgical treatment, it is usually necessary to wait 6–12 months after surgery to assess success (conception) or failure. For older women, their chances of IVF success may have reduced significantly during that time and it may be better for them to move straight on to IVF. Certainly, IVF is appropriate for couples with 2 years or more of infertility with minimal or mild endometriosis. Women with moderate or severe endometriosis may benefit from earlier access to IVF.

The process of an IVF cycle will be described in detail elsewhere. Briefly, treatment involves downregulation of the hypothalamic–pituitary–ovarian axis with GnRH agonist for 2–3 weeks followed by gonadotrophin ovarian stimulation in the 'long protocol', or, gonadotrophin ovarian stimulation with concomitant GnRH antagonist treatment in the 'short antagonist protocol'. Gonadotrophins may either be urinary or recombinant preparations. Once a multi-follicular response is achieved, oocytes are retrieved transvaginally under ultrasound guidance, fertilised in vitro, then cultured for 2–5 days before the trans-cervical replacement of one or two embryos.

An RCT demonstrated that prolonged (3 months) pituitary suppression with GnRH agonist before long protocol IVF in women with endometriosis resulted in a significantly higher live birth rate compared with no pretreatment. A more recent cohort study using prolonged pretreatment with the oral contraceptive pill instead had similar findings. The authors suggested that the prolonged hypothalamic–pituitary axis suppression allowed the 'abnormal' endometrium of women with endometriosis to become normal. The prolonged suppression did not appear to reduce the ovarian responsiveness as the numbers of oocytes retrieved following stimulation were similar in the two groups.

The presence of ovarian endometriosis is associated with a poorer ovarian response and a requirement for a greater total dose of gonadotrophins. However, cumulative live birth rates appear to be similar to those of age-matched controls with normal ovaries. While the presence of endometriomas does not generally impair the results of IVF, it does increase the risk of infection at the time of oocyte collection if the cyst is punctured and may impair access to the follicles. Whether or not endometriomas should be removed before IVF is unclear. Many specialists advise removal of cysts of ≥ 3 cm diameter before IVF, particularly if pain is an issue and if removal may increase the chance of natural conception (that is, satisfactory semen quality and patent fallopian tube[s] are required). Removal will not improve ovarian response during IVF although it may improve access and reduce infection risks. However, since removal requires an operation and involves the risk of causing further damage to the ovary, the decision is unclear in the absence of data from RCTs. Further general disadvantages of IVF include the risk of multiple pregnancy if more than one embryo is transferred, the risk of ovarian hyperstimulation syndrome (OHSS) and the financial expense for the many couples who do not have access to NHS assisted conception funding.

Controlled studies suggest a lower live birth rate for women with endometriosis undergoing IVF compared with women with other diagnoses. However, analysis of very large databases indicates that there is no difference in outcome. It appears that because a comparable number of embryos are available for transfer, even in patients with advanced disease, the outcome of IVF in terms of implantation and live birth rates is similar.

Fertility treatment summary

All couples presenting with failure to conceive should undergo a full evidence-based fertility work-up. This includes a semen analysis, confirmation of ovulation and tubal patency testing. If the semen analysis is abnormal to the extent that IVF with or without intracytoplasmic sperm injection (ICSI) will be required then the tubal check can be avoided. Tubal patency can be tested at laparoscopy or with the use of a hysterosalpingography (HSG) or hysterosalpingo-contrast-sonography (HyCoSy) scan. If women have pelvic pain or signs suggestive of endometriosis, or an endometrioma visible on ultrasound scan, then laparoscopy to test the tubes and diagnose and remove endometriosis disease may be most appropriate. If the fallopian tubes are blocked or there is severe endometriosis disease with adhesions then a rapid move to IVF is indicated. If the tubes are patent and endometriosis is removed then it may be reasonable to allow 6–12 months for spontaneous pregnancy before starting IVF. For women in their late 30s or older and/or who have reduced ovarian reserve suggested on biochemical testing (follicle-stimulating hormone [FSH], antimüllerian hormone [AMH]) and ultrasound [antral follicle count]), an earlier move to IVF may be considered rather than delaying treatment. Prolonged pre-IVF suppression with GnRH agonist or the contraceptive pill is not currently widely used for women with endometriosis. Ovarian suppression does not improve the chance of natural conception.

ENDOMETRIOSIS-RELATED INFERTILITY: KEY POINTS

- Endometriosis is associated with pain and infertility.
- Diagnosis involves visualisation at laparoscopy.
- After a full fertility work-up, expectant management may be appropriate for women with minimal or mild endometriosis.
- There is no place for medical treatment of endometriosis-associated infertility.
- Laparoscopic treatment of minimal or mild endometriosis improves natural fertility.
- Excising, rather than ablating, ovarian endometrioma cysts leads to higher natural conception rates and lower recurrence rates.
- Surgery *may* improve the fertility of women with moderate or severe endometriosis. Assisted conception is often required.
- IVF is appropriate for couples with 2 years or more of infertility associated with minimal or mild endometriosis. Moderate or severe endometriosis may warrant earlier IVF.

Further reading

de Ziegler D, Borghese B, Chapron C (2010) Endometriosis and infertility: pathophysiology and management. *Lancet* 376:730–8.

Giudice LC (2010) Clinical practice. Endometriosis. *N Engl J Med* 362:2389–98.

Jacobson TZ, Duffy JM, Barlow D, Farquhar C, Koninckx PR, Olive D (2010) Laparoscopic surgery for subfertility associated with endometriosis. *Cochrane Database Syst Rev* (1):CD001398.

National Collaborating Centre for Women's and Children's Health, National Institute for Health and Clinical Excellence (2013) *Fertility: Assessment and Treatment for People with Fertility Problems.* 2nd ed. London: Royal College of Obstetricians and Gynaecologists [http://guidance.nice.org.uk/CG156/Guidance].

6 Uterine factors in infertility

Introduction

Uterine factor infertility can be defined as the presence of structural or functional pathology in the uterus that can reduce fertility and diminish the chance of conceiving through assisted reproductive technology (ART) techniques. Embryo implantation, one of the most critical steps in ART, is a complex process that depends on the interplay between the embryo and the endometrium. Surgical management of uterine pathology could therefore be expected to influence the outcome of in vitro fertilisation (IVF) treatment. However, the literature in this regard is largely based on individual experience and observational studies rather than randomised controlled trials (RCTs).

Aetiology

The aetiology of uterine factor infertility can be broadly classified into two categories:

- Congenital uterine anomalies result from a defect in the development or fusion of the paired müllerian ducts. Usually these abnormalities are mediated by a polygenic mechanism, although it is recognised that some occur sporadically.
- Acquired uterine abnormalities include endometrial polyps, fibroids and adenomyosis. Intrauterine adhesions can occur after infections (commonly associated with endometrial curettage, such as following miscarriage or postpartum haemorrhage) or surgery (open or hysteroscopic myomectomy, resection of uterine septum and caesarean section).

Congenital uterine anomalies

The prevalence of congenital uterine anomalies is 6.7% in the general population and 7.3% in the infertile population. The most common anomaly is the septate uterus, with a prevalence of 3.9% in infertile women, followed by arcuate and bicornuate uteri. Women with septate uteri have reduced conception rates and increased risks of first-trimester miscarriage, preterm birth and malpresentation at delivery. The prevalence of arcuate uteri in infertile women is almost identical to that of the general/fertile population (2.1% versus 2.4%). This would suggest that the arcuate uterus does not have a causal role in infertility. However, the findings of a recent systematic review reported an association of arcuate uteri with second-trimester miscarriages. Other defects such as bicornuate, unicornuate and didelphic uterus do not appear to reduce conception rates but are associated with adverse outcomes including second-trimester miscarriage, preterm birth and fetal malpresentation.

It has been suggested that uterine anomalies may contribute to infertility by interfering with normal implantation and placentation. Reproductive outcomes vary according to the type of anomaly and therefore accurate definition and classification is critical.

DIAGNOSTIC MODALITIES

Congenital uterine anomalies are often suspected on two-dimensional transvaginal ultrasound (2-D TVUS) scan. Confirmatory diagnostic tools include 3-D TVUS scan, saline infusion sonography (SIS), hysterosalpingography (HSG), hysteroscopy and laparoscopy. However, these tests have their limitations and none is completely successful in visualising and characterising these anomalies. Table 6.1 outlines the advantages and disadvantages of each diagnostic modality. Pelvic magnetic resonance imaging (MRI) scan has an added advantage of accurately delineating the external and internal contours of the uterus and it also can diagnose the presence of rudimentary horns as well as coexisting urological abnormalities. Although MRI scan is likely to be a relatively sensitive tool, there is a paucity of studies confirming its diagnostic accuracy. In the work-up of a suspected uterine abnormality, a combination of hysteroscopy, laparoscopy, SIS and 3-D TVUS should be considered. Figure 6.1 demonstrates the presence of a sub-septate uterus, and by delineating the external contour of the uterus differentiates it from a bicornuate uterus.

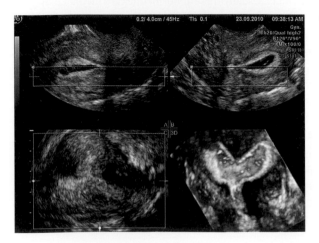

Figure 6.1 A 3-D TVUS scan demonstrating a sub-septate uterus

Table 6.1 Diagnostic modalities in the assessment of uterine pathology

Diagnostic modality	Advantages	Disadvantages
2-D TVUS	• Readily available tool • Cost-effective	• Limited diagnostic accuracy
SIS	• Safe procedure • Associated with lower pain scores compared with other procedures • High sensitivity in diagnostic accuracy • Accurately classifies type, location and size of uterine fibroids, polyps and anomalies	• Potential (low) risk of infection and bleeding
3-D TVUS	• Non-invasive method • Minimal inter-observer variation • Highly reproducible test • High sensitivity and specificity • Can be performed on stored images for future appraisal	• Adequate training in performing the scan and recognition of uterine pathologies is needed
HSG	• Widely available and accepted diagnostic tool • Provides valuable information about the interior of the uterine cavity	• Does not evaluate the external contour of the uterus and therefore cannot differentiate between a septate and bicornuate uterus • Can be a painful or uncomfortable procedure • Associated risks of infection, bleeding and uterine perforation • Exposure to radiation and contrast media • Low sensitivity in diagnosis of intracavitary pathologies
Hysteroscopy	• Considered the gold standard in evaluation of the uterine cavity • Can be used to diagnose and treat intracavitary pathologies simultaneously	• Does not evaluate the external contour of the uterine cavity and cannot differentiate between the various types of anomaly
MRI	• Non-invasive approach • Sensitivity 100% when compared with hysteroscopy and laparoscopy • Added advantage of identifying urological abnormalities	• Expensive • More studies are needed to confirm diagnostic accuracy

HSG = hysterosalpingography; MRI = magnetic resonance imaging; SIS = saline infusion sonography; TVUS = transvaginal ultrasound

CLASSIFICATION OF UTERINE ANOMALIES

The American Society for Reproductive Medicine provided a classification in 1988 that is now the most widely accepted and is used around the world (Figure 6.2).

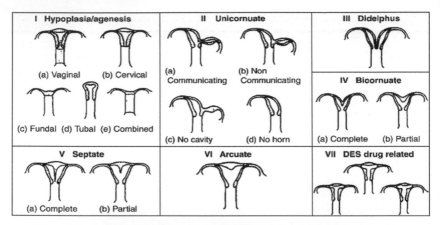

Figure 6.2 Classification of uterine anomalies as described by the American Society for Reproductive Medicine in 1988; reproduced with permission from The American Fertility Society classifications of adnexal adhesions, distal tubal occlusion, tubal occlusion secondary to tubal ligation, tubal pregnancies, müllerian anomalies and intrauterine adhesions. *Fertil Steril* 1988;49:944–55

PROGNOSTIC FACTORS RELEVANT IN DECISIONS FOR SURGERY

It has been argued that, in women with a uterine septum, metroplasty should be considered to reduce the risk of miscarriage and preterm birth. However, there are no RCTs on which to base recommendations. The resection of a uterine septum of < 1 cm in length to improve reproductive outcome is unproven. It has been suggested that surgery for a uterine septum > 1 cm in length may lower miscarriage and preterm birth rates.

There have been no studies evaluating the role of metroplasty in an arcuate uterus to improve reproductive outcomes.

Acquired uterine abnormalities

ENDOMETRIAL POLYPS

Endometrial polyps are one of the most common uterine pathologies. The prevalence of polyps in infertile women scheduled for IVF treatment ranges from 6% to 32% in the literature. The effect of polyps on embryo implantation and therefore on infertility and IVF is uncertain. However, lower conception rates following intrauterine insemination (IUI) in the presence of a polyp have been reported.

Diagnostic modalities

The diagnosis of endometrial polyps can be made by SIS (Figure 6.3), 2-D TVUS or 3-D TVUS (Table 6.1). Polyps appear hyperechoic on a 2-D TVUS scan in contrast to the hypoechoic spongy endometrium during the proliferative phase of the menstrual cycle. In some cases, the endometrium may appear to be bulky and

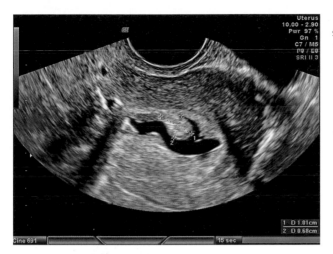

Figure 6.3 An SIS scan demonstrating the presence of an endometrial polyp

disproportionately thick. Application of colour flow can reveal vascularity at the base of the polyp through a feeder vessel. On an HSG, it is difficult to differentiate polyps from myomas or air bubbles. Hysteroscopy is the gold standard for diagnosis of intrauterine polyps and enables their subsequent resection. A systematic review has concluded that SIS and hysteroscopy are equally sensitive in terms of their diagnostic accuracy.

Prognostic factors relevant in decisions for surgery

Polypectomy appears to have a favourable outcome in infertile women. However, it is not clear whether resection of endometrial polyps improves implantation or live birth rates in women undergoing IVF. Polyps are generally resected if the diagnosis is made before the start of IVF treatment, but the evidence supporting this practice is limited. The incidental finding of a polyp during ovarian stimulation is always a dilemma for the clinician, particularly if it is smaller than 20 mm.

INTRAUTERINE ADHESIONS

Intrauterine adhesions may result from infections, previous traumatic instrumentation of the uterus or previous uterine surgeries. Such adhesions are usually composed of dense avascular scar tissue and impede implantation. Patients present with hypomenorrhoea or amenorrhoea.

Diagnostic modalities

Adhesions can be diagnosed by performing SIS or hysteroscopy. The appearances on the SIS scan range from hyperechoic bands present across the uterine cavity to pockets of hypoechoic fluid trapped between the adhesions. The instillation of saline in such cases can cause discomfort to the patient.

Prognostic factors relevant in decisions for surgery

Treatment typically includes hysteroscopic resection of adhesions followed by insertion of an intrauterine contraceptive device (IUCD) (preferably non-medicated) for a period of 6 weeks with additional supplementation of estradiol tablets. Recent literature would suggest that neither IUCD replacement nor estradiol supplementation prevents adhesions or facilitates conception after hysteroscopic resection of adhesions.

UTERINE FIBROIDS

Fibroids are the most common benign uterine tumours, with a prevalence of 5.4–77% in women of reproductive age. Most fibroids are asymptomatic. The mechanism whereby they prejudice fertility is still debated although, intuitively, anatomical distortion and local change in the uterine environment might be expected to affect implantation physiology.

Diagnostic modalities

Fibroid type, location and size can be accurately identified by a routine TVUS (2-D or 3-D) or SIS scan. Fibroids are identified as hypoechoic structures on 2-D TVUS. Ideally, the scans should be performed in the secretory phase, as the endometrium appears hyperechoic in comparison. SIS can readily differentiate polyps from submucosal fibroids irrespective of the phase of menstrual cycle. Furthermore, SIS facilitates surgical decision making by providing information about the precise depth and location of the fibroid within the myometrium. In comparison with SIS, neither hysteroscopy nor HSG has the ability to provide this precise information to aid surgical planning. Figure 6.4 shows the presence of submucosal fibroids on SIS.

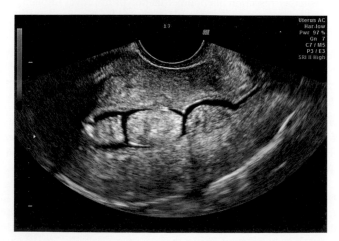

Figure 6.4 An SIS scan demonstrating the presence of a submucosal fibroid

Classification

The European Society of Hysteroscopy classified submucosal fibroids into three grades:

- type 0 describes complete protrusion of a pedunculated submucosal fibroid into the cavity
- type 1 are sessile myomas with less than 50% of the mass in the myometrium, or more than 50% in the uterine cavity
- type 2 are those where more than 50% of the fibroid is within the myometrium.

Treatment options

Adjuvant medical therapy

Gonadotrophin-releasing hormone (GnRH) agonists are sometimes used prior to myomectomy to reduce fibroid size. GnRH agonists may increase preoperative haemoglobin in anaemic patients, reduce uterine and fibroid volume, may enable the use of a transverse incision instead of a vertical laparotomy incision, and reduce intraoperative blood loss. However, there are insufficient data to assess the effects of GnRH agonists on post-myomectomy fibroid recurrence risk and post-operative fertility.

Interventional radiology

Uterine artery embolisation (UAE) successfully reduces fibroid and uterine volumes, and reduces symptoms by 77–86% at 3 months after the procedure. Although there have been successful live births following UAE, the long-term effects of UAE on fertility are uncertain, with reports of premature menopause in the literature.

Surgical options

Observational studies have demonstrated that live birth can follow myomectomy in approximately 50% of patients and that most pregnancies occur within the first 12 months following surgery.

Prognostic factors relevant in decisions for surgery

With regard to IVF treatment, subserosal fibroids do not seem to affect fertility outcomes and thus their removal is not warranted unless ovarian access for oocyte retrieval is impaired. However, if fibroids wholly or partially protrude into the endometrial cavity, decreased pregnancy and implantation rates may be a consequence.

Hysteroscopic myomectomy is now considered the gold standard treatment for submucosal fibroids. An RCT reported a significant improvement in the pregnancy rate in the group of women who had type 0 and type 1 myomas resected.

The impact of intramural fibroids not distorting the uterine cavity (Figure 6.5) on the outcome of IVF treatment remains poorly understood. Recent reviews suggest that IVF-related clinical pregnancy and live birth rates in women with non-cavity-distorting intramural fibroids may be reduced compared with those in women without fibroids.

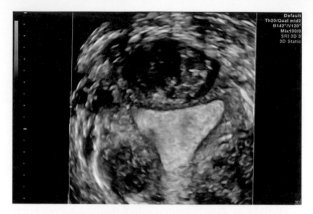

Figure 6.5 A 3-D TVUS image of three intramural fibroids demonstrating that they do not distort the uterine cavity

The dimensions of the fibroid may be an important consideration. One study determined that intramural fibroids larger than 4 cm were associated with a significantly lower pregnancy rate in an IVF cycle. Larger fibroids may have a greater impact on the fertility and reproductive outcomes but well-designed trials are needed to address this important clinical question.

Abdominal myomectomy remains the routine approach for most surgeons faced with multiple or large intramural fibroids. For appropriately trained surgeons, a laparoscopic approach may be adopted. Laparoscopic myomectomy is associated with reduced recovery time, operative blood loss, postoperative pain and overall complications, but with a longer operating time. The literature suggests similar pregnancy rates following either laparoscopic or abdominal myomectomy. Demonstration of reduction in IVF live births in women with non-cavity-distorting intramural fibroids does not necessarily mean that myomectomy will restore live birth rates to the levels expected in women without fibroids.

Existing data do not justify routine myomectomy for all women with infertility. A well-designed multicentre RCT is needed to address this question.

ADENOMYOSIS

Adenomyosis has been linked to poor reproductive outcomes. This is thought to be due to disordered uterine peristalsis and disruption of the myometrial–endometrial junctional zone (JZ).

Diagnostic modalities

An accurate diagnosis can be made with modalities such as MRI and 2-D or 3-D TVUS. The presence of myometrial cysts represents the most specific feature of adenomyosis on a 2-D TVUS scan while the presence of a heterogeneous myometrium is the most sensitive feature. MRI can accurately image the JZ in the uterus, which is thickened in adenomyosis.

In IVF cycles, MRI evaluation of the JZ thickness is the best predictive factor of implantation failure, in that an increase in JZ diameter is inversely correlated to the implantation rate. This observation has important clinical implications as, if the JZ is thicker than 10 mm, it may be necessary to discuss with the patient whether to proceed immediately with IVF or to postpone the procedure and carry out treatment with a GnRH analogue. Early results seem to confirm an improvement of IVF results after this kind of therapy. Attempts to restore fertility in these patients with GnRH agonists coupled with conservative surgery have had minimal success. Other treatments such as UAE and MRI-assisted high-intensity focused ultrasound ablation have been tried with varied success.

Conclusion

Evaluation of the uterus and the uterine cavity utilises a number of investigative tools and is an integral part of the assessment of infertile women. There is a paucity of evidence-based treatment available for some of the uterine pathologies described above. It has been suggested that resection of a uterine septum should be carried out for subfertile patients but there is no robust evidence of benefit. An intrauterine polyp diagnosed before initiation of controlled ovarian stimulation in an IVF cycle should be removed before treatment. The management of polyps diagnosed during stimulation is less clear. Patients with intrauterine adhesions could benefit from hysteroscopic adhesiolysis as this may improve implantation. Hysteroscopic resection of submucosal fibroids before IVF treatment is recommended. Although subfertile women who have otherwise asymptomatic fibroids may benefit from a myomectomy procedure, this approach should be individualised given the absence of any good RCT in this area. The same can be said in the presence of non-cavity-distorting intramural fibroids of more than 4 cm in diameter in women undergoing IVF.

UTERINE FACTORS IN INFERTILITY: KEY POINTS

- Septate uteri are the most prevalent congenital uterine anomaly in infertile women.
- Hysteroscopic metroplasty is a simple and safe procedure but there is a lack of good evidence to strongly recommend it before IVF treatment.
- A polypectomy is advocated before IVF treatment to optimise outcomes.
- Submucosal fibroids (types 0 and 1) can interfere with the implantation process and thus hysteroscopic resection is advocated before assisted reproduction.

Further reading

Chan YY, Jayaprakasan K, Tan A, Thornton JG, Coomarasamy A, Raine-Fenning NJ (2011) Reproductive outcomes in women with congenital uterine anomalies: a systematic review. *Ultrasound Obstet Gynecol* 38:371–82.

Grimbizis GF, Camus M, Tarlatzis BC, Bontis JN, Devroey P (2001) Clinical implications of uterine malformations and hysteroscopic treatment results. *Hum Reprod Update* 7:161–74.

Lieng M, Istre O, Qvigstad E (2010) Treatment of endometrial polyps: a systematic review. *Acta Obstet Gynecol Scand* 89:992–1002.

Pritts EA, Parker WH, Olive DL (2009) Fibroids and infertility: an updated systematic review of the evidence. *Fertil Steril* 91:1215–23.

Sunkara SK, Khairy M, El-Toukhy T, Khalaf Y, Coomarasamy A (2010) The effect of intramural fibroids without uterine cavity involvement on the outcome of IVF treatment: a systematic review and meta-analysis. *Hum Reprod* 25:418–29.

7   Unexplained infertility

Introduction

Infertility is said to be unexplained when standard investigations, including tests of ovulation, tubal patency and semen analysis, are normal. The prevalence of unexplained infertility is approximately 25% but the condition is more commonly diagnosed in women over aged 35 years, indicating that compromised ovarian reserve could be a contributory factor. As standard fertility tests are not comprehensive, they are likely to miss subtle abnormalities in the reproductive pathway, including endocrinological, immunological and genetic factors. The suitability of the term 'unexplained infertility' has therefore been questioned, as it is sensitive to the number, nature and quality of investigations used. However, given the current dependence on assisted reproduction to bypass known and unknown barriers to conception irrespective of cause, it is debatable whether a definitive diagnosis would result in a major change in treatment strategy for many couples.

Management of unexplained infertility

EXPECTANT MANAGEMENT

The decision to treat couples with unexplained infertility should take into account their chances of spontaneous conception, which is affected by female age, duration of infertility and occurrence of a previous pregnancy. The possibility of spontaneous pregnancy in unexplained infertility supports the strategy of expectant management, where couples are advised to continue regular unprotected intercourse in the absence of active medical treatment.

Data from observational studies show that cumulative pregnancy rates associated with such a policy range from 27.4% in a primary care setting to a live birth rate of 14.3% in tertiary care over 12 months. In an observational Dutch study, just over 81% (356/437) of couples with unexplained infertility had an ongoing pregnancy within 5 years of diagnosis, with 74% (263/356) of the pregnancies being conceived spontaneously (Figure 7.1). In a randomised cohort of Scottish women with a mean age of 32 years and a median duration of infertility of 30 months, 17% had a spontaneous pregnancy leading to live birth following 6 months of expectant management. A health economic analysis based on the same trial suggests that an expectant approach is no less cost-effective than empirical clomifene citrate and

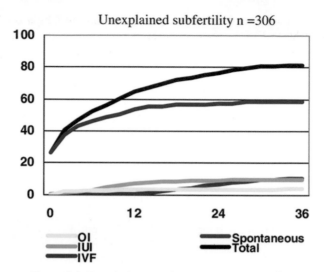

Figure 7.1 Cumulative ongoing pregnancy rates, for 36 months after the first visit, in couples with unexplained infertility; reproduced with permission from Brandes M, Hamilton CJ, de Bruin JP, Nelen WL, Kremer JA (2010) The relative contribution of IVF to the total ongoing pregnancy rate in a subfertile cohort. *Hum Reprod* 25:118–26

unstimulated intrauterine insemination (IUI). Long-term follow up of Dutch couples randomised to a 6-month period of either expectant management or superovulation (SO) plus IUI show similar outcomes in the two groups but an increased cost of €2,616 in those treated actively.

CLOMIFENE CITRATE

The rationale for the use of oral clomifene citrate in unexplained infertility is the belief that it corrects subtle ovulatory dysfunction and encourages the release of more than one oocyte. Treatment is usually initiated with a dose of 50 mg once daily from days 2 to 6 of a menstrual cycle, although higher doses have been used. A transvaginal ultrasound (TVUS) scan is recommended on day 12 in order to identify multiple follicular development, which is associated with a risk of multiple pregnancy. Couples are normally advised to have intercourse from day 12 of the cycle but they are asked to abstain in the presence of excessive ovarian response.

Clomifene is inexpensive, non-invasive and requires little clinical monitoring, but it can cause multiple pregnancies, including high-order multiples. Although recent studies have not confirmed a putative link with ovarian cancer, it is not licensed for prolonged use in the UK. Data from a single large randomised controlled trial (RCT) do not confirm increased live birth rates following clomifene treatment in comparison with expectant management (odds ratio [OR] 0.79; 95% CI 0.45–

1.38). A Cochrane review based on pooled data from this and a smaller earlier trial was unable to demonstrate improved pregnancy rates (OR 1.03; 95% CI 0.64–1.66). Aggregation of data from two trials where clomifene was used together with a human chorionic gonadotrophin (hCG) trigger also failed to show substantial benefit (OR 1.55; 95% CI 0.58–4.60). Data from a single relevant trial suggest that clomifene is less cost-effective than expectant management: the cost per live birth was £72 (95% CI £0 to £206) following expectant management and £2,611 (95% CI £1,870 to £4,166) after empirical treatment with clomifene.

INTRAUTERINE INSEMINATION

IUI has been used widely for the treatment of unexplained infertility. It is thought to enhance the chance of pregnancy by increasing the number of motile spermatozoa within the uterus, bringing them in close proximity to the oocyte. IUI can be performed with concomitant SO, where the availability of more than one oocyte potentially enhances the chance of pregnancy but also increases the risk of multiples.

When IUI in a natural cycle is planned, urinary or serum luteinising hormone (LH) levels are monitored daily from day 10 to day 12 of the treatment cycle and a single IUI is performed 20–30 hours after the detection of an LH surge. Semen is processed by means of either a swim up or a density gradient method and 0.2–1 ml of the prepared inseminate is introduced aseptically into the uterine cavity.

In SO + IUI treatment, clomifene or gonadotrophins are used to encourage ovulation from more than one (ideally two) mature follicles. In clomifene stimulation protocols, a 50 mg oral dose is administered once daily from day 2 to day 6 of the treatment cycle. A TVUS scan for follicle monitoring is planned on day 12. If no endogenous LH surge is detected, an hCG trigger is administered and IUI planned 36–40 hours later.

Where gonadotrophin is used for SO, a dose of 75 iu is administered parenterally from day 3 of a cycle, and follicular growth is monitored by means of TVUS. hCG is administered to trigger ovulation when the leading ovarian follicle measures 17 mm in diameter, and IUI is scheduled 36–40 hours later. To avoid the risk of high-order multiples, cycle cancellation is advised in the presence of more than three follicles measuring more than 15 mm.

In a Scottish multicentre trial that mainly included couples with unexplained infertility, but also contained a small number with mild male infertility and mild endometriosis, live birth rates of 23% (43/191) and 17% (32/193), respectively, were obtained following a strategy of unstimulated IUI versus expectant management over a 6-month period. This difference did not reach statistical significance (OR 1.46; 95% CI 0.88–2.43). The number needed to treat was 17, suggesting that 17 women would need to undergo IUI over 6 months to achieve one extra live birth. A Cochrane review by Veltman-Verhulst et al. was based on this trial with the exclusion of 12% (73/590) of couples with mild male factor infertility and mild endometriosis, thus ensuring that the population only comprised couples with unexplained infertility only. The live birth rate in couples with unexplained infertility randomised to IUI was 23% (38/167), while in those who received expectant management it was 16% (27/167) (OR 1.60; 95% CI 0.92–2.78).

Clomifene + IUI versus expectant management
A Cochrane review pooled data from two trials comparing clomifene + IUI versus expectant management. The results did not demonstrate any evidence of clinical benefit associated with clomifene + IUI (OR 2.40; 95% CI 0.70–8.19) although the wide confidence intervals reflect the uncertainties around this estimate.

SO + IUI versus expectant management
The only study to compare SO + IUI with expectant management in unexplained infertility is a Dutch multicentre RCT. This is also the sole source of data for a Cochrane review that showed that live birth rates associated with SO + IUI and with expectant management were 20% (26/127) and 24% (30/126), respectively (OR 0.82; 95% CI 0.45–1.49). The difference in multiple pregnancy rates between the two arms did not reach statistical significance (OR 2.00; 95% CI 0.18–22.34).

SO + IUI versus timed intercourse in stimulated cycles
A Cochrane review of SO + IUI versus timed intercourse based on data from two trials suggested comparable live birth rates (OR 1.59; 95% CI 0.88–2.88). The combined OR for pregnancy based on data from seven trials was in favour of SO + IUI (OR 1.68; 95% CI 1.13–2.50). The stimulation protocol reported in the studies included clomifene, gonadotrophin and a combination of clomifene and gonadotrophins.

IUI in a natural cycle versus SO + IUI
Aggregated data from four trials indicated that SO + IUI doubles the chances of live birth in comparison with natural-cycle IUI (OR 2.07; 95% CI 1.22–3.50). The relevant Cochrane review on this subject was unable to present a meta-analysis of multiple pregnancy rates as this outcome was missing in some of the primary studies. One of the larger trials reported a multiple pregnancy rate of 29% in the SO + IUI group, compared with 4% in the IUI group.

IUI versus IVF
For couples with prolonged unexplained infertility, there is a general acceptance that assisted reproduction is required but there is some uncertainty about whether to go down the conventional pathway of offering IUI first, followed by in vitro fertilisation (IVF) in those who are not pregnant. In a trial comparing IVF with IUI, differences in live birth rates between IVF (41%) and IUI (26%) were not statistically significant, with an OR of 1.96 (95% CI 0.88–4.36). The wide confidence interval reflects the relative lack of precision of this estimate due to the small sample size.

SO + IUI versus IVF

A Cochrane review by Pandian et al. identified three trials comparing SO + IUI with IVF. Aggregation of data from two of these, which compared three cycles of SO + IUI with one cycle of IVF, did not show a clear difference in outcomes between the two treatments (OR 1.09; 95% CI 0.74–1.59). The multiple pregnancy rates were also comparable (OR 0.64; 95% CI 0.31–1.29).

Data from the third trial could not be combined with the other two owing to statistical heterogeneity. In this trial, 503 couples with unexplained infertility were randomised into two arms. In the first arm women were scheduled to receive three cycles of clomifene + IUI followed by three cycles of SO + IUI followed by IVF; in the second arm women received clomifene with IUI followed by IVF. Pregnancy rates were higher in the second (accelerated treatment) arm (hazard ratio 1.25; 95% CI 1.00–1.56), as were live birth rates (OR 2.66; 95% CI 1.94–3.63).

Results of Cochrane reviews on the effectiveness of various treatments for unexplained infertility in achieving live birth are summarised in Table 7.1.

Table 7.1 Effectiveness of treatments for unexplained infertility (odds of live birth)

Treatment	OR	95% CI
IVF versus IUI	1.96	0.88–4.36
IVF versus expectant management	22	2.56–189.37
IVF versus stimulated IUI	1.09	0.74–1.59
IUI versus expectant management	1.60	0.92–2.78
IUI in stimulated cycle versus timed intercourse in stimulated cycle	1.59	0.88–2.88
IUI in stimulated cycles versus IUI in natural cycles	2.07	1.22–3.50
Stimulated IUI versus expectant management	0.82	0.45–1.49
Clomifene citrate versus expectant management	0.79	0.45–1.38

CI = confidence interval; IUI = intrauterine insemination; IVF = in vitro fertilisation; OR = odds ratio

Cost effectiveness of IUI

A health economic evaluation carried out alongside a multicentre trial found that the cost per live birth for IUI was £1,487 (95% CI £1,116 to £2,155) compared with £72 (95% CI £0 to £206) for expectant management. The authors concluded that IUI was unlikely to be cost-effective in an NHS setting.

Dutch data indicate that the cost per pregnancy resulting in live birth was NLG 8,423 for IUI, NLG 10,661 for SO + IUI and NLG 27,409 for IVF treatment. A British study used a mathematical model to compare the cost effectiveness of primary IVF with IUI and IVF as a treatment option and concluded that a primary strategy of IVF was more cost-effective than IUI or SO + IUI followed by IVF in those who did not become pregnant following their initial treatment.

IVF VERSUS EXPECTANT MANAGEMENT

There are few data from RCTs comparing IVF with expectant management. In a Canadian trial comparing IVF with 3 months' expectant management, the live birth rates were 46% (11/24) in the IVF group (single cycle) and 4% (1/27) in the expectant management group. The difference was statistically significant in favour of the IVF group (OR 22; 95% CI 2.56–189.37).

In an earlier RCT where data on live birth rates were not presented, pregnancy rates for couples with unexplained infertility were 5% (1/21) and 14% (2/14) in the IVF and expectant management group, respectively. The combined OR for pregnancy rate after pooling data from the two trials (OR 3.24; 95% CI 1.07–9.80) was significantly in favour of the IVF group as compared with the expectant management group, although the large confidence intervals reflect the imprecision inherent in these estimates.

Summary

The definition of infertility is based on the expectation of spontaneous pregnancy over an agreed time horizon. It thus essentially represents a prognostic rather than a diagnostic approach to this condition. Data from recent trials have highlighted the role of expectant management in unexplained infertility, and have questioned the effectiveness of empirical clomifene citrate and unstimulated IUI. Although more effective than IUI, SO + IUI is associated with high rates of multiple birth. IVF is used for long-standing unresolved unexplained infertility. As a strategy, it appears to be more effective than SO + IUI in women who have failed to conceive following treatment with clomifene citrate + IUI.

UNEXPLAINED INFERTILITY: KEY POINTS

- Expectant management has a key role in the management of unexplained infertility.
- Empirical use of clomifene citrate is ineffective as a treatment for unexplained infertility.
- Superovulation along with IUI is a more effective treatment than IUI on its own but is associated with multiple pregnancies.
- For couples with prolonged infertility, IVF is an effective option.

Further reading

Bhattacharya S, Harrild K, Mollison J, Wordsworth S, Tay C, Harrold A, et al. (2008) Clomifene citrate or unstimulated intrauterine insemination compared with expectant management for unexplained infertility: pragmatic randomised controlled trial. *BMJ* 337:a716.

Hughes E, Brown J, Collins JJ, Vanderkerchove P (2010) Clomiphene citrate for unexplained subfertility in women. *Cochrane Database Syst Rev* (1):CD000057.

Hunault CC, Habbema JD, Eijkemans MJ, Collins JA, Evers JL, te Velde ER (2004) Two new prediction rules for spontaneous pregnancy leading to live birth among subfertile couples, based on the synthesis of three previous models. *Hum Reprod* 19:2019–26.

Pandian Z, Bhattacharya S, Vale L, Templeton A (2012) In vitro fertilisation for unexplained subfertility. *Cochrane Database Syst Rev* (4):CD003357.

Veltman-Verhulst SM, Cohlen BJ, Hughes E, Heineman MJ (2012) Intra-uterine insemination for unexplained subfertility. *Cochrane Database Syst Rev* (9):CD001838.

8 Assisted reproduction – preparation and work-up of couples

Introduction

This chapter addresses the issues related to patient selection and preparation prior to undergoing assisted reproductive technology (ART) techniques, and the role of regulatory control in ART and welfare of the child assessment. Special aspects of ART including gamete and embryo donation, pre-implantation genetic screening (PGS) and diagnosis (PGD) and fertility preservation are also discussed.

Prognostic factors and patient selection

Age of the female

A woman's age is probably the most significant predictor of successful outcome, and the chances of a live birth after IVF treatment vary considerably with age. The optimal age range for treatment is 23–39 years, with the highest live birth rates being in women under the age of 35 years.

The National Institute for Health and Care Excellence (NICE) fertility guidelines recommend offering three full treatment cycles of IVF to women younger than 40 years who have not conceived after 2 years of regular unprotected intercourse. The use of IVF beyond the age of 40 years is associated with a reduction in the chance of conception and health economic considerations may make the proposition of funding treatment less attractive to those holding budgets for care. Figure 8.1 shows the influence of female age on live birth rates after IVF in the UK.

Duration of infertility

The duration of infertility is also a major factor in determining the likelihood of spontaneous pregnancy. Evidence suggests a significant decrease in age-adjusted live birth rates with increasing duration of infertility between 1 and 12 years.

Ovarian reserve

The number and quality of oocytes decline with a woman's age, as does her overall fertility. Measures to assess the ovarian reserve of oocytes have been used to predict

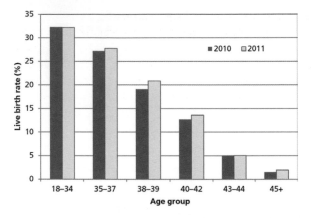

Figure 8.1 IVF live birth rate per cycle started by female age in the UK; data from the Human Fertilisation and Embryology Authority (HFEA)

the likelihood of a successful response to ovarian stimulation with ART treatment. These seem to have a poor correlation with the chance of a live birth. Testing for ovarian reserve is mainly a measure of quantity but may also reflect the quality of oocytes, although the woman's age at the time of treatment is perhaps a better predictor for the latter.

Several tests have been used to assess ovarian reserve. Indirect measurements include early follicular phase follicle-stimulating hormone (FSH) levels, which have been reported to correlate well with the response to ovarian stimulation although the inter-cycle variability is high. Assessment of the antral follicle count (AFC) using ultrasound has also been reported to be an effective predictor of ovarian response. In recent years, measurement of antimüllerian hormone (AMH) has been used in this context with high reported accuracy in assessing ovarian reserve and predicting the response to ovarian stimulation. AMH is produced by the granulosa cells, from the preantral and antral follicles. It can be measured at any time in the cycle and inter-cycle variability is reported to be low. It can also be measured accurately in women receiving hormonal contraception, increasing its practical applicability. Studies have suggested AMH to be equally effective to AFC as a measure of ovarian reserve. The NICE fertility guidelines (2013) recommend the use of one of the following measures to predict the likely ovarian response to gonadotrophin stimulation in women planning to undergo IVF treatment:

- total AFC of 4 or less as a predictor for low response and greater than 16 for a high response
- AMH of 5.4 pmol/l or less for low response and 25.0 pmol/l or greater for a high response
- FSH of greater than 8.9 IU/l for a low response.

Past reproductive history and previous fertility treatment

Women who have achieved a previous pregnancy and particularly those with a previous live birth have a significantly higher live birth rate compared with those with no previous pregnancies. The overall chance of having a live birth following IVF treatment decreases as the number of unsuccessful cycles increases. While the chances of a live birth following IVF treatment are consistent for the first three cycles, the probability of success seems to decrease with subsequent cycles.

Preparation

PATIENT ASSESSMENT AND SCREENING TESTS BEFORE TREATMENT

It is important to obtain a detailed history and to assess couples undergoing IVF carefully before starting treatment in order to allow them to start treatment in their most optimal condition. This will help to identify and manage any medical problems that might prejudice the chance of success as well as pose a risk in pregnancy to mother or child. It is also essential to assess welfare of the child issues, offer counselling and discuss available support options accordingly. Couples should be given information regarding the nature of the treatment and its consequences and risks. They also need to be informed about the measures used for the protection of their personal data and about confidentiality issues. Written consent should be obtained for the use and storage of gametes and embryos and couples should be made aware of their right to withdraw or vary their consent at any subsequent stage.

Women should be offered assessment of their rubella status. Those who are susceptible to rubella need to be offered vaccination and advised not to become pregnant for at least 1 month following vaccination. Screening for *Chlamydia trachomatis* or prophylactic antibiotic treatment should be considered before uterine instrumentation, and enquiry should be made into women's cervical screening history to ensure they are up to date with their screening and avoid delays in starting fertility treatment.

Before the processing of patient gametes or embryos, the couple should be screened for hepatitis B (HBsAg/Anti-HBc), hepatitis C (Anti-HCV Ab) and HIV (HIV-1 and HIV-2, Anti-HIV-1 and Anti-HIV-2) to assess their risk of cross-contamination. Patients testing positive should be offered specialist advice, counselling and appropriate clinical management.

GENERAL HEALTH AND DIETARY ADVICE

Alcohol

Excess alcohol consumption has a detrimental effect on fetal growth and heavy alcohol consumption during pregnancy could result in fetal alcohol syndrome. However, the impact of low or moderate alcohol consumption on the fetus remains uncertain. The Department of Health now recommends that women trying to conceive should avoid drinking alcohol, and during pregnancy women should drink no more than 1–2 units of alcohol once or twice a week. Men should be informed that alcohol consumption within the Department of Health's recommendations of 3–4 units per day for men is unlikely to affect their semen quality, although excessive alcohol intake is detrimental to semen quality.

Smoking
The negative effect of smoking could be due to the effect of nicotine on ovarian, uterine and placental function, resulting in an adverse effect on trophoblast invasion and proliferation. Women should be informed that smoking (or passive smoking) is likely to affect their chance of conception. Men should also be informed that there is an association between smoking and reduced semen quality.

Caffeine
Current evidence does not suggest an association between consumption of caffeinated beverages and fertility.

Body mass index
Women and men with a body mass index (BMI) of more than $29\,kg/m^2$ should be informed that they are likely to have reduced fertility. Women with raised BMI are also at an increased risk of pregnancy loss and complications during pregnancy. A meta-analysis of 16 studies that reported on the association between high BMI and the risk of miscarriage after spontaneous and assisted conception showed that patients with a BMI of more than $25\,kg/m^2$ had significantly higher odds of miscarriage, regardless of the method of conception. On the other hand, the evidence suggests that women with low BMI of less than $19\,kg/m^2$ are likely to improve their fertility chances by increasing their weight.

Folic acid supplementation
Folic acid supplementation is advised before conception and up to 12 weeks of gestation to reduce the risk of fetal neural tube defects. The recommended dose is $0.4\,mg/day$, while a higher dose of $5\,mg/day$ is recommended for women who previously had an infant with neural tube defects or those receiving anti-epileptic medications.

SURGERY FOR HYDROSALPINGES BEFORE IVF TREATMENT
The presence of hydrosalpinx is associated with poor implantation, early pregnancy loss and lower live birth rates. This could be secondary to the toxic effect of the inflammatory fluid within the hydrosalpinx and possible alteration in endometrial receptivity. Surgical treatment should be considered in women with hydrosalpinges before IVF treatment with a view to improve pregnancy rates. Laparoscopic tubal occlusion as an alternative to laparoscopic salpingectomy can be considered.

Further research to assess the value of aspiration of hydrosalpinges before or during IVF procedures and to assess the role of tubal restorative surgery is needed.

FIBROIDS AND INFERTILITY

Studies have demonstrated an association between fibroids and subfertility, although the explanation for this is poorly understood. This association can be related to distortion of the endometrial cavity with submucosal fibroids. Other possible mechanisms include inflammation and alteration of endometrial blood supply resulting in a hostile endometrial environment affecting sperm motility and embryo implantation. Pregnancy outcomes in relation to the location of the fibroids and the effect of surgical treatment on outcomes bear consideration. Women with submucosal fibroids may have lower pregnancy rates and surgical removal appears to improve outcomes. Intramural fibroids appear to decrease fertility, but the benefit of surgical removal in such cases remains unclear. Women with subserosal fibroids have similar fertility outcomes to women with no fibroids and surgical treatment does not appear to alter their outcome. The evidence suggests a less favourable reproductive outcome with uterine artery embolisation (UAE) compared with myomectomy in women with fibroids, and infertility remains a relative contraindication for this procedure.

Regulatory control of ART

In the UK, the regulatory control of ART lies with the Human Fertilisation and Embryology Authority (HFEA), which was established following parliamentary legislation in 1990. It was the first statutory body of its type in the world, and the HFEA's creation reflected public and professional concern about the implications that the new techniques of assisted reproduction might have on human life and family relationships.

The HFEA's principal task is to regulate, by means of a system of licensing, audit and inspection, any treatment or research that involves the use and storage of sperm, eggs and embryos for human application. The HFEA also regulates the storage and donation of gametes (sperm and eggs) and embryos.

WELFARE OF THE CHILD

The HFEA Act states that, before assisted conception treatment is offered, account must be taken of the welfare of any children that may be born as a result of the treatment. It would be expected that medical and physical risks as well as psychological and social factors that could impact on the welfare of the child are considered in this process.

This also covers issues related to growing up in a particular family structure such as single-parent families, same-sex parents, older parents and families in which one or both parents are not genetically related to their children.

Special issues

GAMETE DONATION

Sperm donation

The introduction of intracytoplasmic sperm injection (ICSI) allowed many couples with severe male factor infertility, who would have otherwise resorted to donor insemination, to have their own genetic children. However, there remain a number of situations where donor insemination is indicated, including:

- azoospermia
- infectious disease in the male partner (such as HIV or hepatitis)
- to prevent the transmission of a genetic disorder to the offspring
- severe rhesus iso-immunisation with a homozygous rhesus-positive male partner
- treatment of single women and same-sex couples.

Donor recruitment is performed in accordance with the 2008 UK guidelines for the medical and laboratory screening of sperm, egg and embryo donors. The selection and screening of sperm donors allows the protection of the recipient women from infection and of the offspring resulting from treatment from heritable genetic disorders. The HFEA recommends an upper age limit of 45 years for sperm donors. Donors, in accordance with the HFEA *Code of Practice* (8th edition, 2009, revised 2012), are offered the following screening tests:

- karyotyping
- autosomal recessive disorders (such as cystic fibrosis, thalassaemia and sickle cell disease)
- rhesus antigens
- *Chlamydia trachomatis*
- HIV
- hepatitis B and C
- syphilis.

In the UK, the HFEA *Code of Practice* and the UK guidelines for the medical and laboratory screening of sperm, egg and embryo donors recommend a quarantine period of 6 months for donor sperm before its use to minimise the risk of sexually transmitted viral infections. The HFEA *Code of Practice* suggests an alternative policy for screening sperm donors that could remove the need for quarantining sperm. This consists of viral screening for Ag/Ab testing combined with viral polymerase chain reaction (PCR) (nucleic acid amplification technique [NAT] testing), which may allow treatment to proceed following the initial screening without the need to quarantine donated sperm.

All patients undergoing donor insemination should be offered independent counselling to understand the implications of treatment, both for themselves and for potential resulting children. They need to be made aware of how donors are selected and screened, and of the limitations of accurate matching. The counsellor should also describe the law with respect to the legal position of the child and the parents, and the rules governing confidentiality and anonymity.

The NICE guidelines for the management of infertility recommend that women with no risk factors for tubal disease should be offered tubal assessment after three unsuccessful treatment cycles. Ovarian stimulation is indicated for anovulatory cycles, while, for those with ovulatory cycles, insemination is timed to coincide with ovulation. This is usually determined by daily monitoring of serum luteinising hormone (LH) levels or by a urinary LH detection kit. The live birth rates following donor insemination per cycle started are 15% for women under 35 years and 11% for all ages. Live birth rates following donor insemination decrease with increasing women's age, and women over 40 years have a less than 5% chance of live birth following each donor insemination treatment cycle (UK data from HFEA for 2010).

Egg donation

The main indications for using donor oocytes include the following:

- primary ovarian insufficiency
- bilateral oophorectomy
- irreversible gonadal damage following chemotherapy or radiotherapy
- gonadal dysgenesis associated with Turner syndrome or other chromosomal disorders
- certain cases with a high risk of transmitting a genetic disorder to the offspring
- certain cases of repeated IVF failure, including markedly diminished ovarian reserve, poor-quality oocytes and unexplained failure of fertilisation.

Success rates are primarily dependent on the age of the donor and it is recommended that egg donors should be no older than 35 years at the time of donation. However, with an increasing age of the recipient, there is also a tendency to a slight decline in success rates, possibly due to endometrial ageing. Success rates for IVF using donated eggs have been reported to be similar in women with and without primary ovarian insufficiency.

Before donation is undertaken, oocytes donors should be screened for infectious and genetic diseases in accordance with the guidance issued by the HFEA.

Donors and recipients should be offered independent counselling regarding the physical and psychological implications of treatment for themselves and their genetic children. Careful counselling regarding the potential risks of ovarian stimulation and oocyte retrieval should also be undertaken.

Donors undergo ovarian stimulation as in IVF cycles. The collected oocytes are inseminated with the recipient's partner's sperm and the resulting embryos are transferred into the recipient's uterus. The recipient receives hormone replacement therapy (HRT), using sequential oral doses of estrogens followed by estrogens and progesterones to mimic the natural cyclical hormonal pattern and allow treatment to be synchronised with the donor's stimulation cycle. Recipients who have a spontaneous menstrual cycle require pituitary desensitisation before commencing the HRT regimen, while amenorrhoeic women with ovarian failure do not.

EMBRYO DONATION

Embryo donation may be a suitable option for couples or single patients who require both sperm and egg donation. Both the egg provider and the sperm provider need to be registered as donors, and they need to undergo donor screening to reduce the risk of transmitting diseases or genetic abnormalities to any resultant children. The HFEA *Code of Practice* stipulates that the egg donor should be aged between 18 and 35 years, and the sperm donor between 18 and 45 years. However, in exceptional circumstances, treatment may be carried out using donors outside this age bracket.

DONOR ANONYMITY

Since 1 April 2005, people donating sperm, eggs or embryos in the UK have no longer been entitled to remain anonymous. The change in the law meant that children born as a result of sperm, eggs or embryos donated after that date are entitled to request and receive their donor's name and last known address, once they reach the age of 18. These regulations were not applied retrospectively and, therefore, anyone who had donated before April 2005 is entitled to remain anonymous.

The argument for removal of donor anonymity is based on the right of children born from donated sperm, eggs or embryos to be able to have access to information about their genetic origins, as this may have an important role in the formation of their personal identity. Studies have suggested that concealment of such information could have a detrimental effect on the individual's familial and social relationships, particularly if that information is later discovered in an unplanned manner. It is acknowledged that ending donor anonymity had a negative effect on the availability of donors in the UK since the change in the law was introduced, although research from other countries where anonymity had been removed is reassuring in this respect. In 1985, Sweden changed its laws to allow all donor insemination offspring the right to obtain identifying information about the donor. This resulted in an initial reduction in donors although subsequently the number of donors coming forward returned to the original levels.

SURROGACY

Surrogacy in the UK is regulated under the Surrogacy Arrangements Act 1985 and is carried out within premises licensed by the HFEA. Indications for surrogacy include surgical removal or congenital absence of the uterus and medical conditions such as severe cardiac disease where carrying a pregnancy will impose a significant risk to the health of the woman.

The surrogate will be the legal mother of the child until parenthood rights are transferred to the intended parents through a parental order or adoption after the birth of the child. To obtain a parental order, at least one of the intended parents must be genetically related to the baby (egg or sperm provider). Applications for a parental order must be made to court within 6 months of the birth of the child. Alternatively, if neither of the intended parents is genetically related to the baby (donor egg and donor sperm or donor embryos were used), then adoption of the baby is the only option available to the couple. If the adoption path is used, then a registered adoption agency must be involved in the surrogacy process. The Surrogacy Arrangements Act 1985 and the Human Fertilisation and Embryology Act 1990 permit surrogacy provided that there is no commercial gain as a result of the arrangement.

TYPES OF SURROGACY

Complete surrogacy	Sperm from the partner of the infertile woman is used to inseminate the surrogate mother, who will carry the pregnancy and give the resulting child over to the couple.
Partial surrogacy	The woman has intact ovaries but has an absent or severely malformed uterus. The couple can create an embryo in vitro, then have it transferred to the uterus of the surrogate host.

The ethical aspects of surrogacy are considerable and it is essential that the surrogate host (and her partner) as well as the commissioning couple receive independent counselling and seek legal advice before commencing treatment.

THE PLACE OF PRE-IMPLANTATION GENETIC SCREENING AND DIAGNOSIS

Pre-implantation genetic screening (PGS) involves the assessment of the chromosomal composition of embryos and evaluating for numerical chromosomal abnormalities with a view to selecting euploid embryos for transfer. PGS should be differentiated from pre-implantation genetic diagnosis (PGD), which allows couples where one or both partners carries a known genetic condition to have their embryos tested, to avoid the transfer of a genetically affected embryo. Since its development, the application of PGD has expanded, with over 200 single-gene and chromosomal disorders currently amenable to PGD. It has enabled couples affected by such disorders to avoid the transmission of their genetic conditions to their offspring and avoid the need to undergo prenatal diagnosis.

The risk of implantation failure and pregnancy loss secondary to aneuploidy increases with advanced maternal age, particularly after the age of 35 years. In theory, PGS would allow selection of euploid embryos, and could potentially improve implantation rates and successful outcomes with IVF. However, current evidence does not show improvement in IVF outcomes with PGS, and the routine use of PGS is, therefore, not recommended in women with recurrent implantation failure, recurrent pregnancy loss or advanced maternal age.

There have been a number of explanations as to why PGS could compromise IVF outcomes, despite excluding aneuploid embryos and allowing better embryo selection from a genetic perspective. These include:

- failure secondary to the intervention itself (embryo biopsy, fluorescence in situ hybridisation [FISH] probe fixation and cytogenetic analysis)
- the exclusion of embryos that could potentially develop normally through a self-correcting mechanism within the embryo during the process of embryonic development
- embryo mosaicism – defined as the presence of both anueploid and euploid cells within the same embryo; this has been reported to occur in approximately 57% of embryos biopsied on day 3.

FERTILITY PRESERVATION

Sperm cryopreservation

Sperm cryopreservation should be considered for men with conditions that are likely to impair fertility such as malignancies and for those about to receive chemotherapy or radiotherapy. This provides an opportunity to preserve fertility and for the sperm to be used for assisted fertilisation at a later date. The evidence suggests no decline in sperm viability with time and thus that there is no biological time limit to cryopreservation.

Oocyte cryopreservation

Cryopreservation of oocytes has a lower success rate compared with cryopreserved embryos. This technique has been used for women with conditions that are likely to impair fertility (cancer/chemotherapy/radiotherapy) and for fertility preservation – 'social egg freezing' in women wishing to preserve their fertility potential. Over 1000 live births have been reported following fertilisation of cryopreserved oocytes.

Recent systematic reviews have shown higher oocyte survival rates in vitrified oocytes compared with slow-frozen oocytes. The fertilisation rate, embryo cleavage rate and rate of good-quality embryos were also all higher with oocyte vitrification. Vitrification appears to be an efficient method to preserve oocytes, but there is a need for more large controlled clinical trials to strengthen this conclusion. In clinical practice, at present, there has been a gradual shift towards the use of vitrification in this context.

Ovarian tissue cryopreservation

Cryopreservation of ovarian tissue followed by auto-grafting or in vitro culture has been suggested and may be a valuable option in conserving fertility. This, however, is still at an early stage of development and more research is needed to explore this area.

Cryopreservation of ovarian tissue allows the storage of a large number of primordial and primary follicles and holds the promise of providing a larger pool of oocytes for future use in such groups of patients. This can be performed using slow-freezing techniques or vitrification, with recent studies suggesting a better outcome with the use of the latter in this context. The clinical application and use of the cryopreserved ovarian tissue, however, remains a challenge. Auto-transplantation of cryopreserved cortical fragments is currently the only available option in clinical practice that allows the use of the cryopreserved tissue, although with a low success rate, and 20 reported live births with this technique to date. In vitro maturation of the oocytes will probably provide a more promising application, although studies on animal and human primordial oocytes obtained using this technique are at an early stage, and not near clinical application.

Conclusion

The process of assisted reproduction is complex and may result in significant physical and emotional stress for the couples undergoing treatment. It is, therefore, important to assess couples carefully to ensure that they start treatment in their most optimal state and to identify and manage any medical problems. It is also essential to assess for welfare of the child issues to try to determine the couple's ability to look after a child, and to offer counselling and discuss available support options accordingly.

The evidence assessing ovarian reserve tests overall shows good prediction for the response to ovarian stimulation but seems to have poor correlation with pregnancy outcomes. The response achieved with gonadotrophin stimulation during an ART treatment cycle may well be the best indicator of a woman's ovarian reserve, while her age is a good predictor of oocyte quality and the chances of a successful treatment outcome.

ART – PREPARATION AND WORK-UP OF COUPLES: KEY POINTS

- Success of fertility treatment is affected by the woman's age, duration of infertility and previous pregnancies.
- The regulation of fertility treatment in the UK is undertaken by the HFEA, which was established following the Human Fertilisation and Embryology Act 1990.
- The evidence assessing ovarian reserve tests overall shows good correlation with response to ovarian stimulation but poor prediction for pregnancy outcomes.
- Salpingectomy should be offered to women with hydrosalpinx before IVF treatment as this improves the chances of pregnancy and live birth.
- Surgical removal of submucosal fibroids improves pregnancy rates. Intramural fibroids are associated with lower pregnancy rates, although the benefit of surgery in such cases remains unclear.

Further reading

National Collaborating Centre for Women's and Children's Health, National Institute for Health and Clinical Excellence (2013) *Fertility: Assessment and Treatment for People with Fertility Problems.* 2nd ed. London: Royal College of Obstetricians and Gynaecologists [http://guidance.nice.org.uk/CG156/Guidance].

Human Fertilisation and Embryology Authority (2009, revised 2012) *Code of Practice.* 8th ed. London: HFEA [www.hfea.gov.uk/docs/8th_Code_of_Practice.pdf].

Association of Biomedical Andrologists; Association of Clinical Embryologists; British Andrology Society; British Fertility Society; Royal College of Obstetricians and Gynaecologists (2008) UK guidelines for the medical and laboratory screening of sperm, egg and embryo donors (2008). *Hum Fertil (Camb)* 11:201–10.

World Health Organization (2010) *WHO Laboratory Manual for the Examination and Processing of Human Semen.* 5th ed. Geneva: WHO [http://whqlibdoc.who.int/publications/2010/9789241547789_eng.pdf].

9 Assisted reproduction – clinical and laboratory procedures

Introduction

Assisted reproductive technology (ART) includes all treatments that involve in vitro handling of human gametes (oocytes and sperm) and embryos to establish a pregnancy. It is estimated that over 3.75 million babies have been born worldwide using ART since 1978 following the birth of the first in vitro fertilisation (IVF) baby, Louise Brown. Although ART is used synonymously for IVF, other techniques involving gamete manipulation (Table 9.1) have also been used, for the most part before routine use of IVF, and they are rarely used now.

Table 9.1 ART techniques used in the past

Procedure	Description
Gamete intrafallopian transfer (GIFT)	Oocytes and sperm are placed in the fallopian tube under laparoscopic/hysteroscopic guidance.
Zygote intrafallopian transfer (ZIFT)	Oocytes are collected and fertilised in vitro; the resulting zygote is then placed into the fallopian tube.
Peritoneal oocyte and sperm transfer (POST)	Oocytes and sperm are transferred to the pouch of Douglas.

As IVF is the most common ART procedure in current use, it is the focus of this chapter. The process includes stimulation of ovaries with gonadotrophins followed by oocyte collection, fertilisation in vitro in the laboratory and subsequent embryo transfer within the uterus (Figure 9.1).

Controlled ovarian stimulation

PHYSIOLOGY OF THE HYPOTHALAMIC–PITUITARY–OVARIAN AXIS IN A NATURAL CYCLE

In a natural cycle, selection of the dominant follicle is established in the first 5–7 days and consequently peripheral levels of estradiol begin to rise significantly by day 7.

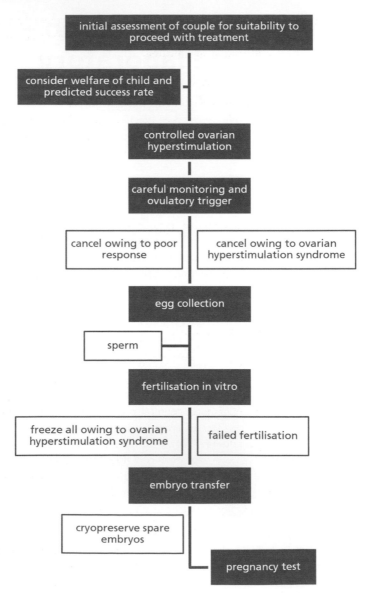

Figure 9.1 Summary of an IVF treatment cycle

These levels gradually increase and exert a progressively suppressive influence on follicle-stimulating hormone (FSH) release. At the same time, rising estrogen exerts a positive influence on luteinising hormone (LH) secretion. The LH surge initiates the continuation of meiosis in the oocyte, luteinisation of granulosa cells and synthesis of progesterone within the follicle. Progesterone enhances the activity of proteolytic enzymes responsible, together with prostaglandins, for digestion and rupture of the follicular wall, leading to ovulation.

OVARIAN STIMULATION IN AN ART CYCLE

ART cycles generally seek to produce multiple oocytes in order to obtain several embryos and thus facilitate choice in the selection of embryo for transfer, maximising the chance of a successful cycle. It is usually necessary to stimulate the ovaries with supraphysiological doses of gonadotrophins.

Gonadotrophin stimulation

Choice of gonadotrophins

For a while there has been a debate in the literature as to which gonadotrophins are best: urinary gonadotrophins (human menopausal gonadotrophin [hMG]) or recombinant FSH. However, the latest evidence suggests there is no difference in live birth rate or ovarian hyperstimulation rate in the two types. It is recommended that the clinical choice of gonadotrophin should depend on availability, convenience and cost.

Factors influencing dose of FSH

The daily dose of gonadotrophins depends on ovarian reserve. The aim of stimulation is to produce an adequate number of oocytes without hyperstimulation. Initial starting doses of FSH are 112.5, 150, 225 and 300 iu. Some practitioners have employed doses as high as 600 iu per day but there is no evidence that increasing the dose to this level increases the live birth rate. In fact, there are recent concerns that higher dose leads to recruitment of more aneuploid oocytes. In young patients with good ovarian reserve, 150 iu should be sufficient; in older women and/or those with poor ovarian reserve, a higher dose (300 iu) is needed. There are suggestions that women who are overweight or obese require 20% higher doses of gonadotrophins. In those with polycystic ovaries, the dose of gonadotrophins has to be very carefully titrated as there is a very narrow therapeutic window between over- and under-response; these patients are usually commenced at the dose of 150 iu.

Minimal stimulation IVF

There is increasing interest in the application of milder stimulation protocols that aim to render IVF treatment more patient-friendly, reduce the chance of complications (especially ovarian hyperstimulation syndrome [OHSS]) and lower costs. Good success rates have been described. In minimal stimulation regimens, 150 iu of FSH is commenced from day 5 of stimulation instead of day 2 as is usually the case with conventional regimens.

Natural cycle IVF

Another variation is natural cycle IVF, where no gonadotrophin stimulation is used. Instead, the woman's own cycle is used, which will usually develop only one oocyte per cycle. Natural cycle IVF is hampered by high cancellation rates due to premature LH rises or premature ovulation and has reduced chances for successful oocyte retrieval. The planning of oocyte retrieval based on an LH rise requires frequent monitoring and round-the-clock oocyte retrieval and laboratory facilities.

Pituitary suppression

While there is a need to produce multiple oocytes, the challenge is to do so without dangerous overstimulation. When multiple follicles grow, there will be a rise in estrogen and consequent negative feedback on the pituitary gland thereby decreasing FSH, which will prevent further follicular growth. Moreover, with high estradiol levels there is risk of a premature LH surge that could disrupt normal follicle and oocyte development, making treatment less successful. It is therefore important to suppress endogenous pituitary activity so that multiple follicles can develop. There are two different types of agent used for pituitary suppression, both analogues of hypothalamic gonadotrophin-releasing hormone (GnRH). The preparations used are either GnRH agonists or antagonists (Figure 9.2)

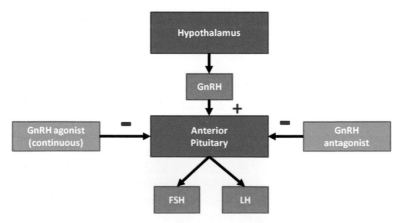

Figure 9.2 GnRH analogues used in IVF

GnRH agonists

Continuous GnRH agonist exposure causes gonadotrophin suppression via pituitary desensitisation after a transient period of gonadotrophin hypersecretion – the flare effect. Pituitary suppression takes at least 7–10 days to establish. Use of GnRH agonists improves success rates compared with stimulation with gonadotrophins alone. Various regimens of GnRH agonists have been described in the literature.

Long protocol

The long protocol involves the administration of GnRH agonist for at least 14–18 days to achieve maximal suppression of ovarian activity before commencing gonadotrophin administration. There are two types of long-protocol regimens. The long follicular protocol involves the use of GnRH agonist from the first day of the cycle, and the long luteal protocol starts GnRH agonist administration from the mid-luteal phase of the previous cycle. In both, the gonadotrophins are commenced after at least 2 weeks of GnRH agonist. The agonists are continued up until the day of the last dose of gonadotrophins, which is usually the day of human chorionic gonadotrophin (hCG) administration – the ovulatory trigger.

Other variations used in long-protocol regimens include the cessation or reduction of agonist exposure at the start of stimulation or mid-way during stimulation. This is based on the principle that the suppressive effect of agonists lasts for at least 10–12 days. There is no difference in clinical pregnancy rates with either of these variations.

Short protocol
In short-protocol treatment cycles, the GnRH agonist is started at the same time as gonadotrophins – day 2 of the menstrual cycle. GnRH agonist is continued up until the last day of gonadotrophin injections – the day of hCG administration.

Ultra-short protocol
The ultra-short protocol uses only the initial flare effect of the GnRH agonist. GnRH agonist is commenced a day before gonadotrophin injections and is given only for 3 days. Gonadotrophins are continued alone after that. These regimens are usually recommended for those patients in whom a suboptimal response to gonadotrophins is expected; they are sometimes referred to as predicted poor responders.

There is evidence of a significant increase in clinical pregnancy rate (OR 1.50; 95% CI 1.16–1.93) with the long protocol as compared with the short protocol. GnRH agonist can be given by either depot injection or daily subcutaneous injections, or by nasal spray. There is no difference in the live birth rate comparing daily or depot injection. However, the amount of gonadotrophins required to elicit a satisfactory ovarian response increases with the use of depot preparation. There has been wide variation in the dose of GnRH agonists used, ranging from 100 to 1000 µg/day.

GnRH antagonists
GnRH antagonists compete directly with endogenous GnRH for receptor binding and therefore rapidly inhibit secretion of gonadotrophin and steroid hormones. Unlike agonists, antagonists produce immediate profound suppression of LH; that is, within hours of administration. The time duration of treatment is thus shortened. Gonadotrophins are started on day 2 of the cycle, followed by the antagonist on day 6 or when the leading follicle reaches a diameter of 14 mm, whichever is earlier. The most commonly used dose for GnRH antagonist administration is 0.25 mg. A recent meta-analysis has shown that the live birth rates are similar whether the agonist or antagonist regimen is used. In addition, there is a significant reduction in the risk of OHSS when antagonists are used. However, the planning of cycles can be more difficult when the antagonist is used for pituitary suppression. To circumvent this, pretreatment with the oral contraceptive pill has been suggested.

This increases the duration of treatment, which is an argument against routine use of antagonists. However, for those who are at risk of OHSS and have limited time (for example, oncology patients), antagonists are the treatment of choice. Recent data have proven the safety of antagonist regimens.

A recent worldwide survey has shown that agonist long protocols are still the most common regimen in use, and the uptake of antagonists is only 12.1% cycles worldwide (www.ivf-worldwide.com/survey/survey-the-use-of-gnrh-agonist-in-ivf-protocols-results.html). There is, however, a shift towards using GnRH antagonist regimens because of the advantages mentioned above.

Cycle monitoring

Monitoring of treatment includes follicle tracking with ultrasound (Figure 9.3) and ovarian steroid measurement. There is no evidence from randomised trials to support cycle monitoring by ultrasound plus serum estradiol as being more efficacious than cycle monitoring by ultrasound alone, using outcomes of live birth and pregnancy rates as comparators. The reasons for monitoring are to identify women at risk of ovarian hyperstimulation early in stimulation and to reduce their dose. Sometimes treatment has to be cancelled even before reaching the oocyte collection in the interests of safety.

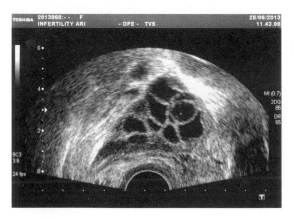

Figure 9.3 Multiple follicular development during controlled ovarian stimulation for IVF

Ovulatory trigger

HUMAN CHORIONIC GONADOTROPHIN

hCG is the most commonly used ovulatory trigger. Once the follicles are mature, hCG is given to facilitate final maturation of the oocyte. Oocyte retrieval is usually scheduled 34–36 hours after administration of hCG. During this time, cytoplasmic changes take place within the oocyte, meiosis is resumed, and the intercellular cytoplasmic connections between granulosa cells and the oocyte are interrupted.

Prophase of the first meiotic division is resumed and the oocyte progresses to metaphase of the second meiotic division.

GnRH AGONIST

GnRH agonist is sometimes used as the ovulatory trigger to prevent excessive follicular development in women at high risk of developing OHSS. The agonist can only be used where antagonists are used for pituitary suppression. Routine use is not recommended for all cycles as they are less effective than hCG in terms of the live birth rate per randomised woman (OR 0.44; 95% CI 0.29–0.68).

Oocyte retrieval

PROCEDURE

In the early days of IVF, oocyte collection procedures were done under laparoscopic guidance. The advent of transvaginal ultrasound-guided aspiration techniques rendered the procedure simpler, safer and more efficient. Vaginal ultrasound is used to visualise the maximal diameter of each follicle, allowing the needle to enter the centre of each follicle. Normally, a single puncture is needed to reach all the follicles in a single ovary. A pedal-operated suction pump with a vacuum regulator is used. The maximum aspiration pressure is set at $-15\,\mathrm{kPa}$ or $-125\,\mathrm{mmHg}$.

Various kinds of needle are used; usually, a 17 gauge single lumen needle is used when no flushing is required. In the presence of more than four follicles, follicular flushing has not been shown to improve live birth rates.

ANALGESIA/ANAESTHESIA

The use of analgesia and anaesthesia varies among clinics, with some using conscious sedation and others using short general anaesthesia. A recent UK survey revealed that the majority of units (84%) used intravenous sedation for transvaginal oocyte collection, whereas 16% used general anaesthesia.

COMPLICATIONS

Transvaginal ultrasound-guided oocyte collection is a relatively safe procedure. However, there is a small risk of complications.

Infections
There is a very small risk of infection. Prophylactic antibiotics are administered to avoid this.

Bleeding
There is a small risk of bleeding following oocyte collection from the vaginal wall puncture site. Control is usually achieved with the application of pressure on the site of bleeding, Suturing is rarely required. If the internal iliac vessels are accidentally punctured, laparotomy is required in the presence of active bleeding.

SPECIAL CIRCUMSTANCES

Hydrosalpinx

Removal of hydrosalpinges before commencing treatment is associated with improved success rates. However, if for any reason a hydrosalpinx is detected for the first time during stimulation or at oocyte collection, or the patient is not suitable for surgery, it is reasonable to continue with treatment. One should not aspirate the hydrosalpinx during the procedure of oocyte retrieval as it contains toxic fluid that is harmful for the oocytes. Given that success rates almost halve in the presence of a hydrosalpinx, it may be advisable to freeze the embryos, remove the hydrosalpinx and transfer thawed embryos at a future date. For women unsuitable for surgery, the hydrosalpinx may be aspirated at the end of the procedure and oral antibiotics should then be given for 5–7 days.

Endometrioma

Ideally, endometriomas should have been dealt with before starting stimulation. However, not all endometriomas need surgery. At the time of oocyte collection, one should avoid puncturing an endometrioma because the viscous content blocks the needle. In addition, this is associated with a higher risk of infection. If an endometrioma is punctured at oocyte retrieval, the patient should be given oral antibiotics for 5–7 days.

High ovary on transvaginal ultrasound

Most ovaries become vaginally accessible after stimulation. If, at the time of oocyte retrieval, the ovary remains high, it is sometimes the case that the application of abdominal pressure renders the ovary accessible by the vaginal approach. Occasionally, it may be necessary to consider a laparoscopic oocyte retrieval if the ovaries are adherent to the lateral pelvic wall.

In vitro maturation of oocytes

In vitro maturation (IVM) involves the growth of immature oocytes (at the germinal vesicle stage) in culture up to the metaphase II stage after their earlier retrieval from the ovaries, thus reducing the risk of OHSS. Observational studies have shown oocyte maturation rates of up to 80.3%, fertilisation rates of up to 76.5% and clinical pregnancy rates of up to 50% per cycle.

Laboratory procedures

FERTILISATION

After oocyte retrieval, freshly ejaculated seminal fluid is prepared to concentrate motile spermatozoa in a fraction that is free of seminal plasma and debris. Embryologists then have to decide whether they are going to perform conventional IVF or need to inject sperm directly into the oocyte (intracytoplasmic sperm injection [ICSI]).

Conventional IVF

Insemination is usually performed 40 hours after hCG administration, with each oocyte inseminated with 50 000–200 000 motile spermatozoa. For conventional IVF, all oocytes that are obtained are inseminated. There is no need to clean the oocytes before insemination. It is suggested that the granulosa cells surrounding the oocytes serve to provide an environment for further maturation of the oocytes, if they were slightly immature. The cells also play a role in natural sperm selection.

ICSI

ICSI was first introduced in 1992 for severe male factor infertility. Since then it has revolutionised the treatment of male infertility throughout the world, as it has been possible for men with azoospermia and very severe oligoasthenozoospermia to have their own genetic child. ICSI is used in up to 60% of all reported ART cycles. The indications for ICSI are:

- low count and or low motility
- vasectomy reversal (due to presence of antisperm antibodies)
- previous failed fertilisation
- previous low fertilisation
- sperm obtained by surgical sperm retrieval techniques.

Although ICSI was initially used for male factor infertility, it has also been widely used for various other indications such as:

- low number of oocytes
- older women
- mild male factor infertility.

Before carrying out ICSI, the oocytes have to be cleaned and denuded of all surrounding cells. The mature oocytes (metaphase II), are then selected and injected with a single sperm (Figure 9.4).

Fertilisation and early embryonic development

The rate of normal fertilisation after conventional IVF is about 60% per inseminated oocyte. Fertilisation rates with ICSI are around 80% per injected oocyte. Insemination is performed 40–42 hours after hCG administration. Thereafter, following an incubation/injection period of 16–18 hours in culture medium, oocytes are examined to ensure that normal fertilisation, as defined by the presence of two pronuclei, has occurred. Cell division ensues, usually reaching the four-cell stage by day 2 and the eight-cell stage on day 3.

About 5% of oocytes fail to fertilise, and this generally attributed to impaired sperm–zona interaction. Another 5% cases exhibit abnormal fertilisation, which could be due to polyspermy or non-extrusion of the second polar body. Such embryos are not suitable for transfer. Embryos are maintained in culture within an

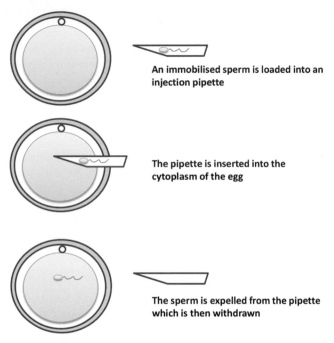

An immobilised sperm is loaded into an injection pipette

The pipette is inserted into the cytoplasm of the egg

The sperm is expelled from the pipette which is then withdrawn

Figure 9.4 Intracytoplasmic sperm injection (ICSI) into a denuded metaphase II oocyte

incubator at a constant temperature of 37° C and a humid atmosphere containing 5% CO2. Currently, most laboratories use snapshot assessment of embryos at various times to select the best embryo to transfer. More recently, time-lapse imaging techniques have been developed that allow continuous monitoring of embryos; they also provide potentially useful information about the dynamics of embryo development and may assist in embryo selection. Table 9.2 shows the typical timing of observations of fertilised oocytes and embryos, and the expected stage of development at each time point.

In some laboratories, an additional check for early cleavage is done at 26–28 hours after insemination as the time and pattern of the first cell cleavage of the zygote has been shown to predict both embryo quality and implantation.

The gradual attrition in numbers at each stage from fertilisation through cleavage-stage divisions to blastocyst should be noted. Approximately 30% of fertilised oocytes are good-quality blastocysts on day 5.

EMBRYO TRANSFER

It is essential that high-quality embryos are selected for transfer to maximise the chance of conception. Embryo selection can be achieved in a number of ways and a variety of scoring systems have been developed that take account of embryo

Table 9.2 Timing and purpose of checks for early development of embryos

	Hours after insemination	Name	Purpose/importance
First check	17 ± 1	Pronucleus (PN) check	To check fertilisation and detect abnormal fertilisation (normal fertilisation is associated with the observation of two pronuclei within the cytoplasm)
Second check	44 ± 1	Day 2 check	To determine the cleavage; it is expected that the best embryos will be at the four-cell stage
Third check	68 ± 1	Day 3 check	To (1) check further development; (2) decide whether extended culture is suitable; (3) select the best embryo to transfer on day 3; (4) select the embryos to freeze.
Fourth check	116 ± 1	Day 5 check	To determine the best embryo to transfer and select the embryos to freeze; embryos should be at blastocyst stage by this time

development at key stages of embryogenesis. Developmental milestones that are considered are described in Table 9.2.

If only one oocyte is fertilised, embryo transfer can be performed on day 2 (day 0 being day of oocyte collection). If two or more embryos are available then culture to day 3 is usually recommended and the best single embryo may be selected for transfer at that point. If enough good-quality embryos are present on day 3 and it is difficult to choose the best one, extended culture to day 5 is advised. This is based on the principle that chromosomally normal embryos will self-select themselves and poor-quality ones will fail to reach the blastocyst stage. Moreover, the transfer of embryos at the blastocyst stage (day 5) could be considered to be more physiological as this is similar to the time of implantation in spontaneous conception.

Embryos are placed within the endometrial cavity just below the fundus of the uterus, using a soft catheter. Pregnancy rates per blastocyst transfer can be as high as 60%. If embryo transfer is carried out under ultrasound guidance, a higher ongoing pregnancy rate can be achieved as compared with non-ultrasound-guided transfer (OR 1.38; 95% CI 1.16–1.64).

LUTEAL PHASE SUPPORT REGIMENS

Adequate luteal phase support is recommended during IVF and ICSI to maximise implantation and pregnancy rates. This can be achieved by substituting deficient LH with GnRH agonists or with hCG (which has a longer half-life), or directly by using progesterone with or without estrogen.

A recent Cochrane review showed a significant positive effect of progesterone for luteal phase support, favouring synthetic progesterone over micronised progesterone. The addition of other substances such as estrogen or hCG does not seem to improve outcomes. Progesterone is typically given for 2 weeks, although in some centres it is continued up to 12 weeks of gestation. Various routes of progesterone administration can be considered – intramuscular, oral, rectal or vaginal – although here is no convincing evidence that a specific route or duration of administration is better than another. The use of hCG for luteal phase support is associated with a higher risk of OHSS.

CRYOPRESERVATION

Cryopreservation is used in a number of circumstances, as discussed below.

When extra embryos are available

If, after embryo transfer, good-quality spare embryos are available, couples are usually offered cryostorage of the surplus embryos. There are two methods of cryostorage: slow-freezing and vitrification. Vitrification is a relatively recently introduced ultra-rapid freezing method that may reduce the threat of damage from ice crystal formation such as can occur in slow-freezing. Better thaw-survival rates have been claimed with this technique as compared with slow-freezing.

Sometimes, if sperm cannot be obtained on the day of oocyte collection, oocytes need to be frozen. Vitrification is the preferred method for freezing oocytes, and good fertilisation rates post-thaw can be achieved. ICSI rather than conventional IVF is needed post-thaw.

Prevention of OHSS

When a large number of oocytes are generated, there is a risk of ovarian hyperstimulation. It is sometimes recommended to patients that all embryos should be frozen, allowing their use later in a natural or hormone replacement regulated cycle. Deferring embryo transfer in an overstimulated fresh cycle reduces the risk of developing OHSS and, where hyperstimulation does occur, it may be of a milder nature. With a fresh transfer, where pregnancy ensues, OHSS if it occurs tends to be more severe and associated with serious morbidity.

Fertility preservation in oncology patients

Cryopreservation of embryos or oocytes is used before chemotherapy to preserve fertility. When there is no partner available, oocytes are vitrified after going through the process of ovarian stimulation and oocyte collection.

Fertility preservation for social reasons

As more women delay childbearing, with improved techniques of cryopreservation, some women are freezing their oocytes for use in later life. Although, this technique is well accepted for oncology cases, there is a lot of controversy when used for social reasons.

Factors affecting IVF success rates

Although the average live birth rate after IVF/ICSI treatment is around 25%, success is dependent on various factors: the age of the woman, the duration of infertility, previous reproductive history, obesity and smoking. Of these, the age of the woman is the single most important predictor of success, with the chances of success declining as female age advances (Figure 8.1).

Consequences of treatment

Two major complications of ART to consider are multiple pregnancy and OHSS.

MULTIPLE PREGNANCIES

Initially to improve the success of ART, multiple embryos were transferred, resulting in a surge in the prevalence of twins and higher order multiple births. In recent years, regulatory policies encouraging the transfer of embryos singly have led to a dramatic reduction in the number of high-order multiple pregnancies. However, in the UK in 2010 nearly one-quarter of ART conceptions were still twins.

Single-embryo transfer is now advocated as the default embryo transfer practice in many countries and this has led to a marked reduction in these countries in the incidence of ART twins. Although elective single-embryo transfer (a policy of transferring a single embryo when more than one are available) is the only way to reduce the multiple pregnancy rate, there is a wide variation in the global uptake of this technique, with multiple social, economic and clinical factors being responsible.

OHSS

OHSS is an iatrogenic complication of ovulation induction and ovarian stimulation for ART and is characterised by cystic enlargement of the ovaries and rapid fluid shifts from the intravascular compartment to the third space. It is a potentially life-threatening condition in its severe form. hCG, either exogenous or endogenous, is the triggering factor of the syndrome. The relationship between hCG and OHSS is thought to be mediated via the production of angiogenic vascular endothelial growth factor (VEGF).

OHSS presenting within 9 days of the ovulatory dose of hCG is likely to reflect excessive ovarian response and the precipitating effect of exogenous hCG, while OHSS presenting after this period reflects endogenous hCG stimulation from an early pregnancy. This is poorly correlated to ovarian response. Late OHSS is significantly more likely to be severe and to last longer than early OHSS.

Certain women are at higher risk of OHSS, such as those with a history of previous OHSS, those with polycystic ovary syndrome, younger women, those with a low body mass index (BMI), and women exhibiting a high number of follicles and/or high estradiol levels during stimulation and who conceive.

Diagnosis of OHSS is based on the history and the symptoms. Account should be taken of factors such as:

- the degree of ovarian response following stimulation
- abdominal distension
- abdominal pain

- nausea and vomiting
- dyspnoea.

Most cases of OHSS can be managed on an outpatient basis, with oral analgesics and patient advice with respect to indicators of worsening illness that may necessitate more aggressive intervention. A review every 2–3 days for many patients is likely to be adequate. Urgent clinical review is necessary if the woman develops increasingly severe pain and abdominal distension, shortness of breath or a subjective impression of reduced urine output. If the woman conceives, prolonged monitoring may be required. Symptomatic relief of moderate OHSS with an anti-emetic and stronger analgesics should be accompanied by careful monitoring, including physical examination, ultrasound and weight measurement, and laboratory determination of haematocrit, electrolytes and serum creatinine, ideally on a daily basis. In non-conception cycles, mild or moderate OHSS is likely to resolve spontaneously after menstruation. However, in patients who become pregnant, rising levels of endogenous hCG significantly increase the risk of developing severe OHSS.

With the advent of ovarian reserve assessment using measures of antimüllerian hormone (AMH) and antral follicle count (AFC), patients at high risk of OHSS can be identified and gonadotrophin stimulation regimens can be adjusted to take account of this. Mild stimulation, natural cycle IVF and the use of in vitro maturation (IVM) are strategies aimed at reducing this complication.

ART – CLINICAL AND LABORATORY PROCEDURES: KEY POINTS

- IVF is used synonymously with ART.
- ICSI is the most common method of fertilisation in IVF practice around the world.
- There are various stimulation regimens to choose from.
- The day of embryo transfer depends on the number and quality of embryos.
- Progesterone is the best agent for luteal phase support.
- Multiple pregnancies are a potential hazard of ART and limiting the number of embryos to be transferred will diminish this risk.
- Age of the female partner is the most important predictor of successful outcome.

Summary

The use of IVF has radically transformed the way in which we approach the management of infertility, irrespective of the diagnosis, and it is integral to the infrastructure of a modern fertility service. Factors affecting prognosis have to be considered carefully in determining whether any treatment offered carries a realistic chance of success. In addition, the potential for complications, some of which can be life-threatening for the woman, should be borne in mind.

Further reading

National Collaborating Centre for Women's and Children's Health, National Institute for Health and Clinical Excellence (2013) *Fertility: Assessment and Treatment for People with Fertility Problems.* 2nd ed. London: Royal College of Obstetricians and Gynaecologists [http://guidance.nice.org.uk/CG156/Guidance].

Nyboe Andersen A, Carlsen E, Loft A (2008) Trends in the use of intracytoplasmatic sperm injection marked variability between countries. *Hum Reprod Update* 14:593–604.

Brown J, Buckingham K, Abou-Setta AM, Buckett W (2010) Ultrasound versus 'clinical touch' for catheter guidance during embryo transfer in women. *Cochrane Database Syst Rev* (1):CD006107.

Child TJ, Abdul-Jalil AK, Gulekli B, Tan SL (2001) In vitro maturation and fertilization of oocytes from unstimulated normal ovaries, polycystic ovaries, and women with polycystic ovary syndrome. *Fertil Steril* 76:936–42.

Alpha Scientists in Reproductive Medicine and ESHRE Special Interest Group of Embryology (2011) The Istanbul consensus workshop on embryo assessment: proceedings of an expert meeting. *Hum Reprod* 26:1270–83.

Index

Page numbers in *italics* refer to figures or tables